# Table of Contents

# *FREE BONUS!!!*

**Hi! This is Adam Trainor, author of _The Diet Myth_ and founder of www.SoundBodyLife.com**

I want to thank you so much for taking the time to read this book- these simple tools have had a huge impact on my life, and I hope that they will change your life too!

If you'd like to get updates about future books, and a special FREE GIFT delivered straight to your inbox, just click the link below!

All it takes is an e-mail!

## *Send me my free bonus now!*

Enjoy the book, and thanks again!

Adam

# The Diet Myth: Mistakes that are Making You Fat and the Simple Secrets to Losing Weight and Keeping it Off

## Introduction

"A new year, a new you." How many times have we heard that phrase? Every January, thousands of people decide that enough is enough and that it's time to start another new diet in the hopes that we'll lose some weight. We set a target, whether it's a birthday, a holiday, or another important event, and decide exactly how much weight we want to lose between now and then.

Then we start with rock solid motivation and dedication. Typically, just under half of us will have fallen off the dieting wagon completely by the third month. Those of us who do make it to their target weight will rejoice at our success, but for many of us, it will be short lived as we will then revert back to our old eating habits and the weight will start to creep back on.

The term diet comes from the Greek word *dieta,* which means 'manner of living'. However, for most of us, when we think of the word diet we immediately think of a temporary way of eating. Diets are considered to be short-term changes to both what we eat and the way we eat it—a means to an end. We think of them as a quick fix and this is only encouraged by some of the more extreme diet regimes, which make sensationalist claims and take advantage of our impatient nature.

What they neglected to share is how unsustainable these regimes are in the long term, as well as the possible damage these diets actually do to our bodies in the end. As humans, we need to eat for health, not just for weight loss, and we are going to explain why.

Within this eBook, we're going to look at the concept of dieting and why the fad diets that we see advertised are *not* the solution to the problem. We will consider what our bodies need to create a healthy *and* a sustainable diet—a true manner of living. Exploring the makeup of our food and drink, how to read between the lines of product descriptions, and the responsibilities of those in charge of both manufacturing and selling the products will all help you to make an informed decision as to what constitutes a healthy diet. We will get you moving with advice on how to incorporate exercise into your diet in such a way you won't even realize you are doing any!

Finally, we will help you process all this information by giving you tips on what you need to do to get started including: planning, shopping lists, sample recipes, and links to helpful resources. You have taken the first step just by reading this introduction. You don't have to rush to understand everything at once. Take it one section at a time and before you know it, you will have a made the changes needed for a truly healthy lifestyle.

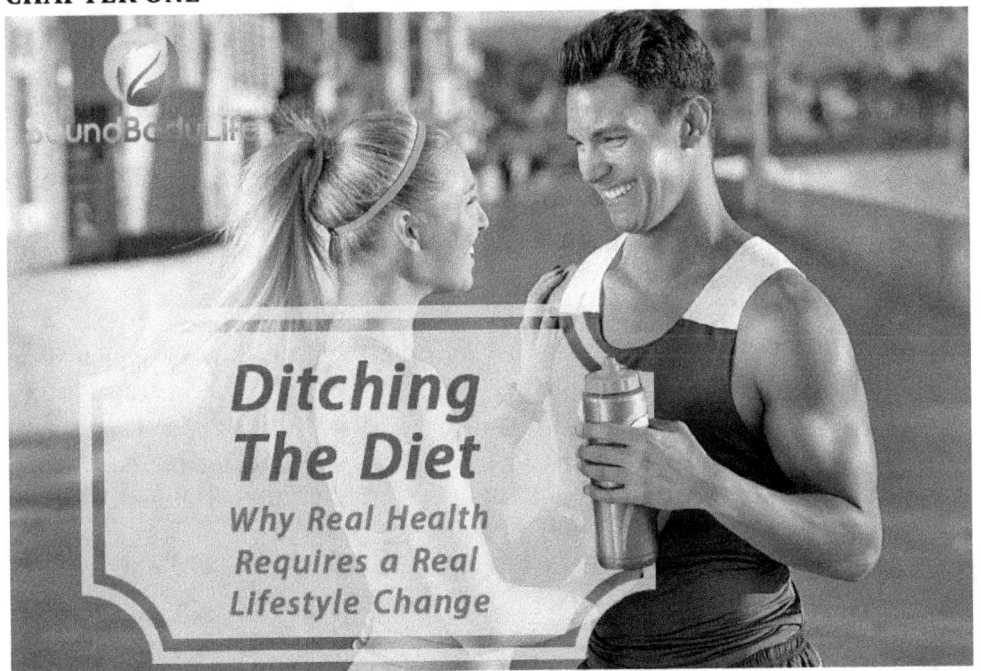

# CHAPTER ONE

## Is food really the problem?

Many of us that suffer from obesity may not realize that food may not be the actual problem, but a symptom of it. People tend to fall into two categories during times of extreme emotion: those who over eat and those who don't eat anything at all. Eating is linked to our emotions, as the use of our gut and digestive system kicks our neurotransmitters into life. It also produces serotonin, which is responsible for balancing our moods. As such, it may be that there are other factors influencing our weight and causing us to eat for comfort. Emotional eating is very common and in order to begin change to our weight, it is necessary to identify and solve the emotional changes causing us to eat in the first place.

## Why dieting isn't the solution

As we have said, dieting is not the solution. Not only does dieting implicate only a temporary change, but it focuses specifically on food consumption. Granted, yes, food is a vital part of maintaining good health and combating obesity, but it is certainly not the only key to an overall healthy lifestyle.

WebMD lists over 100 different diets on its website, everything from the "African Mango Diet" to the "Zone Diet". Many of these diets will certainly help you lose weight, at the very least in the short term, but are they truly healthy? Take for example, "The Cabbage Soup Diet". "The Cabbage Soup Diet" only markets itself as a week-long diet that should not be followed for any longer. You can eat as much of the food on the prescribed list as you like during that time which basically includes: fruit, vegetables, and a very tiny amount of carbohydrates or proteins.

Oh, and a lot of cabbage soup! It's a very high-fiber and low fat eating plan which can see you lose up to ten pounds during that time. However, participants in the diet have claimed side effects such as: dizziness, nausea, headaches, weakness, and bloating during just that one week of dieting. This is because their bodies are suffering through the lack of proper nutrition. The first week of eating normally after the diet usually results in constipation and some weight gain. So yes, while you may initially lose a large amount of weight, you are also doing your body considerable damage in the process.

A recent study of people followed after successfully losing weight via a diet found that a staggering 83% of them gained back more weight than they had initially lost. This is a phenomenon commonly known as 'weight cycling'. Studies have shown that weight cycling is not just ineffective, but has the potential to damage your health in the long run. Professor Mann, a psychologist at the University of California (UCLA), analysed 31 long-term studies that followed individuals on a variety of diets that lasted between two and five years. Her research, which was then published in American Psychologist magazine, concluded that people would be better off not dieting whatsoever rather than repeatedly doing so—as yo-yoing in size was putting strain on the body. Other studies have illustrated a link between repeatedly gaining and losing weight and a number of serious cardiovascular diseases, diabetes, stroke, and altered immune function.

The regain of weight lost through dieting shouldn't really be considered a surprise. With the temporary nature we associate with dieting, comes the point whereby we reach our goal or milestone. When this happens, we believe that we can then go back to eating as we did before, which is undoubtedly principally unhealthy foods and far too much of it. Another psychologist at UCLA talking about the long-term study on dieting stated that, "One of the best predictors of weight gain.... was having lost weight on a diet at some point during the years before the study started", which is a frighteningly accurate prediction.

## Why fasting is dangerous

Fasting is becoming a popular way of either kick-starting or maintaining weight loss. The 5:2 diets are especially well known, whereby the dieter eats what they want within reason for five days of the week and adheres to a strict 500 calorie intake on the other two days. The two days can be together, apart, or changed to be flexible to your needs. It sounds relatively easy in theory, but the main issue is that those who follow the diet tend to still consume far too many calories on the normal days. It also doesn't change the way we think about food, instead it just limits what we can have on certain days. However, the 5:2 diets are just the tip of the iceberg when it comes to fasting diets.

Whilst medical evidence supports the fact that intermittent fasting is a sure fire way to kick-start weight loss or beat specific cravings, does it not then follow that long-term fasting could be even more beneficial?

## Long-term fasting

There are a number of varieties of long-term fasting. The most frightening and extreme of them have been termed a 'dry fast' during which you may not consume *anything* at all, not even water. This is beyond dangerous. Your water intake should match if not exceed the water that we excrete every day. This is why we are advised to drink at least two to three litres of fluid every day to maintain our water balance and kidney function. Dehydration has a number of serious side effects, progressing from dizziness and drops in blood pressure to damage to our internal organs and even death.

Other types of long-term fasting diets include: 'water fasting', which allows for the consumption of water only during the time of the fast and no calories whatsoever. Another technique is 'juice fasting', which lets the dieter drink only fruit and vegetable juices. Some people also fast on bone broths or extremely low-calorie protein supplement and water mixes. While these are not technically fasts as they do allow a very small amount of calories into the body, they are both still highly dangerous and in particular protein fasting, as our bodies were not designed to live on protein with no accompanying fats.

## What does a long-term fast mean for my body?

It is obvious that the biggest benefit of long-term fasting is quick weight loss. With nothing coming in and out of your body, but still using calories to function day to day, the weight will begin to shed very quickly. During the first 24 hours of a fast, your body uses all of the glycogen in your liver. This is transformed into glucose to give us energy. Once this has been depleted, the body will be forced to burn protein or fat to get energy. So, for the first few days of a fast, you can expect to shed one to two pounds per day through water loss and initial protein-burning before your body switches to stored fats.

It doesn't sound too bad yet, does it? Stored fats are the preferential source to break down to create energy, being more energy-dense per pound than protein. At this point, weight loss slows a little—down to a pound approximately every two days. Your body finds it a little more bearable as being in ketosis (fat burning) begins to suppress your hunger anyway. However, after the initial burning of stored fat, your body will switch back to protein to convert to energy too, protein that has been pulled directly from your muscles. It will do this even if there are stored fats still available. What if I told you that your body isn't picky about which muscles it breaks down? You can't choose to lose a little off your biceps or gluts. All of your major muscles become affected, including your heart. Fasting puts undue stress on your heart by cannibalizing your cardiac muscle for fuel. That's right; it eats away at your heart muscles causing damage and a risk of heart failure.

Water fasting also creates a risk of heart failure due to the lack of minerals in your diet. Potassium and Magnesium are especially necessary for cardiac function and you cannot get these through water alone. During the 1950s and 60s, fasting was used experimentally as a way to treat obesity. It had fatal consequences with several patients dying from heart failure.

Your heart isn't the only thing at risk from fasting. Your immune system becomes compromised, putting you more at risk of infectious diseases that your weakened body may not have the energy to fight. Other less serious side effects include: mood swings, general irritability, low energy, and dizziness caused by low blood pressure.

Like with most crash diets, fasting and extreme fasting are effective ways to rapidly lose a good amount of weight, but some weight gain is inevitable once you begin to eat normally again. Real and sustainable weight loss requires one thing: real and sustainable change!


**Creating change, one step at a time**

We have identified that we need to completely alter our lifestyle in order to combat our weight demons, defeat addictions, and achieve real health. This can be a daunting prospect, but it *is* achievable.

## Start Small!

Start by making one small change per day. A simple swap of a chocolate bar to a piece of fruit or swapping fizzy drinks for water is a good example.

## Get motivated!

Some people suggest sticking a "fat" picture on their fridge to remind them of how they don't want to look, but health isn't about outer beauty. Looking at a picture of you overweight and an unhappy self will only serve to remind you of the negative feelings you felt at that time. Instead, put a picture on the fridge of yourself when you felt at your best as to help stay positive and create an emotional connection with what you are striving towards.

## Get support!

Supportive family and friends are invaluable during the first few weeks and months of change. Explain to them why it is so important to you to take these steps. Truly supportive people will not dangle temptation in front of you. For a night in at a friend's house, suggest you all take a dish that you like, that way you can ensure to take something that won't compromise your healthy eating regime. Don't just stop with friends and family though. Medical support is just as important. Speak to your doctor and see if there is a local mentoring program that you can be a part of.

## Make time!

One of the most common excuses for poor eating habits and a lack of exercise is that people struggle to make time to do these things. Eating properly and healthy will require preparation time, so get organized. By always having something healthy prepared, you have no excuse not to make the right choices.

Keep a large bowl of mixed salad in the refrigerator, the fruit basket stocked, and a large bottle of water chilling. When you cook your meals, you can always make a little extra and freeze it so you have a quick, healthy, and nutritious dinner that only needs to be zapped in the microwave.

## Changing your eating habits

Changing the *way* we eat is just as important as changing *what* we eat. Some of our habits can be good, but many can be bad. For example, 'I always have dessert'. Sudden changes to our eating habits are often ineffective and harder to stick to. One popular method used to alter eating habits is known as the 'Three R's'.

# Reflect

Look at all your current eating habits, both the good and the bad, and identify any triggers you may have for unhealthy eating. Keeping a food diary may be the best way to help you do this. Writing down how you feel each time you reach for food may also help identify any emotional eating triggers such as: sadness, stress, or fatigue.

Common weight-gaining habits include:
- Skipping meals, particularly breakfast
- Eating when not concentrating i.e. watching TV or playing video games
- Always cleaning your plate
- Always eating desserts
- Eating while travelling i.e. in the car or on a train or bus
- Eating when not hungry

Eating when you're not hungry is more common than you think. It is very easy to be tempted by: opening the fridge, candy at grocery store checkouts, or someone in the office passing around cakes. Boredom is also a huge cause of eating when we are not hungry, but just feel that we should be doing something. Clue—eating is not it!

Once you have identified some of your unhealthy eating habits, make sure that you understand what the triggers are that cause them to occur. This is vital to making the change and will act as cues to warn you of these triggers ahead of time. Select the few that you would most like to work on first, for example: mid-afternoon fatigue that has you reaching for sugar-filled snacks.

# Replace

This really is as simple as swapping your unhealthy eating habits for good ones or avoiding the situation altogether. For example, swap from eating in front of the television to eating at the table. The lack of distraction will allow you to focus on your meal and you'll realize sooner when you're full. Other ideas can include: making time for breakfast, swapping a mid-morning muffin for a fruit salad, or planning an activity for times when you know boredom usually sets in.

Once you have alternatives in place for replacing your unhealthy habits, they will in time become second nature to you.

## Reinforce

There will be times that you may fall off the wagon, but the important thing is to get back on it again and remind yourself as to why you are making this journey to a healthier lifestyle. Habits take time to break and replace. There is real skill in being able to pull yourself back after a slip and return to your new lifestyle, rather than 'blowing off' the whole day or, even worse, the whole week.

## Next Steps to Success

This chapter has taken a look at unhealthy eating, why dieting doesn't work, and why extreme diets, like fasting, are actually dangerous to your health. We have explored why the very word diet suggests a short term solution to what actually needs to be a lifelong dedication to proper and sustainable health.

Finally, we have looked at identifying triggers for unhealthy eating habits and some basic steps that we can take to both prepare for and overcome these in order to make new, healthy choices for both our bodies and mind. By reading this chapter, you have indicated that you want to make the change and we are going to help you every step of the way.

In the next chapter, we are going to delve a little deeper into the world of those naughty little things called calories which make our clothes tighter. Also, we are going to explore a number of different foods and drinks to examine why they aren't good for us. Being well informed is vital when it comes to changing to a truly healthy lifestyle. Are you ready to know more?

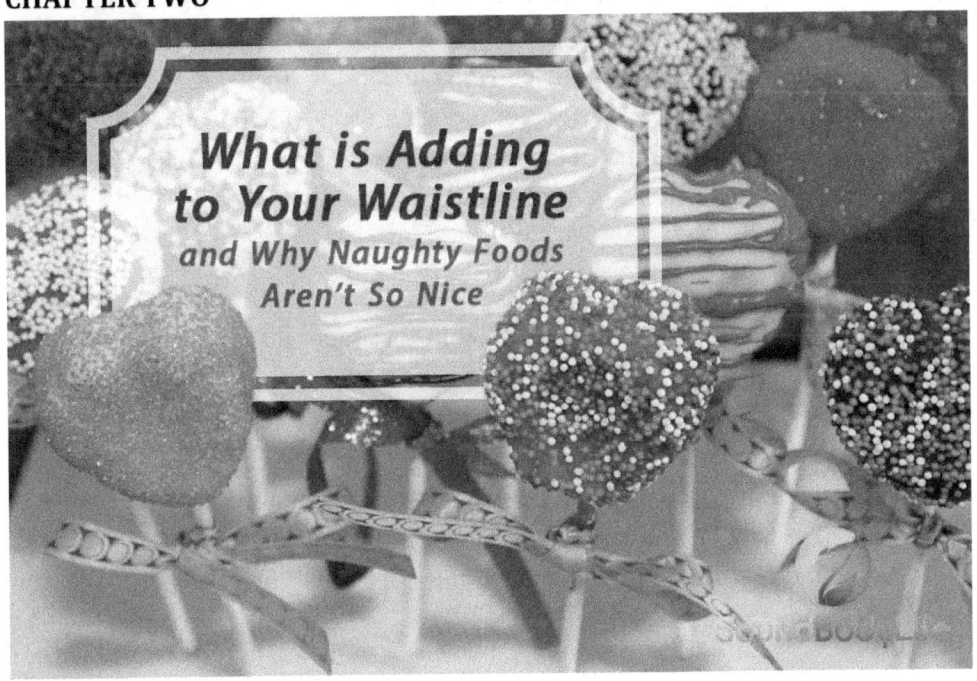

# CHAPTER TWO

# What is Adding to Your Waistline
### and Why Naughty Foods Aren't So Nice

During this chapter, we are going to take a look at calories: what they are and what they mean for us. We will, also, consider what makes specific foods unhealthy.

## What are Calories?

Calories are a fundamental element in the composition of our food and drink, on a par with protein or minerals, and are tools of measurement just like inches, ounces, or liters. Their function is to measure the amount of energy that is in your food or drink from the fat, protein, carbohydrates, and alcohol that it contains. One calorie is the equivalent to 4.184 joules of energy. If we were to say something contains 100 calories, this would describe how much energy our bodies could expect to receive from consuming it. Our bodies consume calories every minute of every day. Even breathing requires energy!

The more strenuous the impact is on our bodies, the more calories we will use. This is also the case when fighting an illness. Our bodies have to work harder to fight the illness and maintain all of the usual functions. This means additional energy is required in order to have the energy to work as hard as it needs to.

Foods and drinks contain a mixture of both calories and nutrients, and it is essential to get the right combination of the two in our diet. Foods that are considered to be 'bad' for us typically have far too many calories and not enough nutrients. Nutrients are the components found in food that our bodies use to grow and survive. They include: amino acids, lipids, and carbohydrates. Let's examine some nutrients in more details.

## Carbohydrates

The optimum diet is suggested to contain between 80 and 100 grams of carbohydrates every day, which are obtained from foods like vegetables, whole grains, milk, and meat. This works out to around 60% of our daily diet. Our bodies turn carbohydrates into glucose, which we then use for energy. However, carbohydrate quality is important and some sources of this vital nutrient are better than others. For example; it is much better to get carbohydrates from unprocessed, natural food rather than manufactured meals and soda drinks.

## Proteins

The basic building blocks of protein are a chain of amino acids. While some amino acids can be made by our bodies, other essential ones must be found in our diets. These are most commonly found in fish, meat, poultry, milk, beans, and cereal grains. Proteins are needed in order to both grow and repair our cells efficiently. Proteins are rarely used for energy unless there is a lack of carbohydrates, in which case some muscle proteins are broken down. Also, excess protein can be used for energy or it is sometimes converted to fat.

## Fats

Fats, technically known as lipids, provide the best source of energy for us to function. Fatty acids are an essential component of them that we are unable to make for ourselves and these are commonly found in some food sources including: nuts and seeds, olives, avocados, and peanuts. Although fat is vital to the function of our body, there are many problems caused by consuming an excessive amount. With this in mind, it is critical to try and maintain a balanced intake.

## Vitamins

Vitamins are something that our body is unable to make for itself and they are required in small amounts for it to work efficiently. They are organic molecules that promote metabolic reactions and varying vitamins can be found in all of our food sources. Fat-soluble vitamins such as A, D, K, and E are stored in our liver and fatty tissue for future use. This means that they are not required by the body on a daily basis. However, others, for example: Vitamin C and B Vitamins, are not stored in the body and need to be consumed more frequently. They are known as water-soluble vitamins. They are organic molecules that promote metabolic reactions and varying vitamins can be found in all of our food sources.

## Minerals

Minerals are required in small amounts to help our body to function. They are especially useful for controlling body fluids inside and outside cells, assist in turning our food into energy, and building strong teeth and bones. Essential minerals: such as calcium and iron, can be found in copious foods including fruit, vegetables, dairy products, meats, and fish.

Studies have linked imbalances to various diseases and serious medical conditions including diabetes, hypertension, and even cancer. Controlling the proportions of calories and nutrition in your diet is a crucial part of changing to a healthy lifestyle.

## Diet Drinks – Dispelling the Myth

When trying to lose weight, many people swap their usual soda for diet versions of the same drink. Almost every major brand of sugar-sweetened beverage has a 'diet' version of it. However, instead of being laden with sugar, they are sweetened with artificial sweeteners like Aspartame, Saccharin, Sucralose, Cyclamate, and Acesulfame K. We are tempted by labels stating that these diet versions are 'calorie-free' or 'sugar-free' and so we immediately think that they will be a healthy alternative. Drinks that are calorie-free mean that in theory you should be able to lose weight while drinking them and they should prevent against the development of sugar-related diseases like diabetes.

*Myth: Calorie-free and sugar-free beverages are healthy choices.*

*Fact: Unless followed by other positive lifestyle changes, choosing diet drinks over regular ones will have absolutely no impact on your health and wellbeing.*

The reality is that there is evidence that links diet beverages to a number of serious health concerns, some of which we will examine in a little more detail.

## Diet drinks and Diabetes

The Diabetes Association ([www.diabetes.org](www.diabetes.org)) reports that over 30 million American citizens now have diabetes, with almost 95% of them being diagnosed with Type II, which is particularly common in obese individuals. In 2010, diabetes was listed as the seventh leading cause of death in the United States, with 234,051 death certificates naming diabetes as an underlying or contributing cause to death. Also, there are countless other conditions associated with it including: hypoglycaemia, high blood pressure, stroke, blindness, and amputations to name just a few. Scary, huh?

Diabetes is one of several major diseases directly linked to sugar consumption, so it would be reasonable to suggest that replacing sugar laden drinks with a sugar-free variety would be beneficial. However, there is no evidence to support this theory whatsoever. In fact, quite the opposite is true. One study of 66,118 French women followed them for a total of 14 years and found that those who had consumed the largest number of diet drinks had a 121% greater risk of developing Type II diabetes. Other data analysis from two studies by Harvard concluded that diet drinks raised the risk of diabetes in women by 6% for each daily serving.

In our opinion, there is no sustainable benefit to swapping to diet beverages and research suggests that they may actually be detrimental to our health.

## Diet drinks and Obesity

As we have said, the switch to diet drinks is often made because of a desire to lose weight and cut back on the calories. We mistakenly believe that zero calories means that we can consume as much of that product as we like with no effect. Or if we don't consume any calories in our drinks, then we can have second helpings or an over- indulgent dessert. In our minds, zero calories equals healthy and this is really not the case.

In San Antonio, Texas, a study of 3,682 people showed double the risk of obesity in those who drank diet versions of beverages. Another controlled trial showed that drinking diet soda had no conclusive effect whatsoever.

Unfortunately, there is very controversial evidence regarding the links between diet drinks and obesity. However, what we can be certain of is that cutting calories from one part of your life does not necessarily mean that you can consume them in another part!

### Diet drinks and Metabolic Syndrome

Metabolic Syndrome is the name for a combination of obesity, high blood pressure, and diabetes, which while dangerous to your blood vessels in their own right, when combined become deathly hazardous. It is defined by having the following factors present:

- A waist circumference of over 31.5 inches for women and over 37 inches for men
- Consistently high blood pressure (140/90mmHG or above)
- Insulin resistance
- High cholesterol
- An increased risk of deep vein thrombosis or other blood clots
- A tendency to develop inflammation of body tissue

You could be forgiven for believing drinking sugar free or calorie free drinks would help reduce the risk of developing Metabolic Syndrome. In theory, it should. However, there is no evidence to support this. One study saw 9,514 people were followed for nine years and the report, published in 2008, reported that artificially sweetened beverages were associated with a 34% increased risk of developing Metabolic Syndrome.

In our opinion, there is no significant support to suggest that drinking diet beverages may be effective in preventing the development of Metabolic Syndrome.

Most of the studies that we have looked at here are what is known as epidemiological studies, which examine patterns, causes, and effects of health related conditions. This means that they can only show links and associations rather than conclusive results. In our opinion, there is very little to support the consumption of any form of diet beverage and, as such, if you truly want to drink something healthy and completely risk free, swap to water!

**Artificial Sweeteners—not so sweet?**

Saccharin was the first artificial sweetener discovered in 1879 by a chemistry research assistant by the name of Constantine Fahlberg. Since that time, a number of others have been discovered and they are now utilized in hundreds of products across the globe, as well as being readily available to add to your own cooking or beverages.

The American Heart Association (AHA) and American Diabetes Association (ADA) have cautiously given some mild support to the use of artificial sweeteners instead of sugar as a way to help in the fight against obesity, diabetes, and other similar diseases and it is easy to see why. Offering the sweetness without the calories, artificial sweeteners appear to be an ideal road to effective weight loss. To give you an idea: the average 12oz can of sugar-sweetened soda contains around 150 calories, with almost all of them coming from sugar. If you were to drink the equivalent of three cans of soda per day, not an unreasonable amount of fluid, you would expect to consume 450 calories per day just in your choice of drink. That is approximately a quarter of the recommended daily amount of calories for the standard healthy weight range female, or one fifth for men.

As we have said, many people feel that by cutting out calories in one way means that they are then free to consume them in another. We fool ourselves into thinking that it is okay to have an extra slice of pizza because we are drinking a diet drink. Some research shows that artificial sweeteners can over stimulate our sugar receptors, which may limit our ability to tolerate more complex tastes. In other words, naturally sweet foods may not taste sweet enough and we may dislike savoury tastes entirely, instead craving artificially flavoured foods with much less nutritional value. Also, there has been research that points to certain addictive tendencies shown by people who consume a number of diet drinks per day. Animal studies of rats that were exposed to cocaine and then given a choice between the drug and an artificial sweetener reported that the majority of the rats opted for the sweetener.

While the FDA has ruled the use of artificial sweeteners to be safe, the studies used to come to this decision were based on much smaller consumptions than is currently seen today. With this in mind, there is really no way to know what effect large amounts of artificial sweetener will have on our bodies either now or in the years to come. So the question is: would we be better off sticking to sugar? Well, the answer really depends on what form that sugar comes in. Natural sugars, such as the sort found in fruit, are relatively healthy as it is packed with nutrients, high in fiber, and has a low glycemic load. In comparison, refined sugars, also called refined carbohydrates, have had much of their organic goodness removed, making them unhealthy and lacking any nutritional benefit.

## So what's the deal with refined carbohydrates?

One definition of the term *refined* is 'processed,' which accurately describes the way in which refined carbohydrates are created. Examples of refined carbohydrates include: food products made with white flour instead of whole grain, such as white bread and pasta.

## What do refined carbohydrates do to my body?

The best illustration of the effect of refined carbohydrates comes in the form of paper-Mache paste. The traditional way to make paper-Mache paste involved mixing white flour with water to form a stodgy, sticky substance that would act as a glue to hold the newspaper in place. Imagine spooning that paste into your mouth and eating it. As it makes its way down your digestive system, it hardens more and more, making it incredibly difficult for your body to break down. It sits in your stomach like cement, leaving you feeling uncomfortable and bloated. Well, this is what happens when we eat refined carbohydrates like white bread. When the bread, which is made with white flour just like the paper-Mache paste, becomes moistened with our saliva, it becomes just like that paste. There is nothing in it to help us to digest it, no nutrients to absorb to benefit from; it is just a mass of starch. Not a nice thought is it?

Refined foods are basically a shell of the natural product that they should be. Fiber, bran, minerals, and vitamins have all been removed. While this process increases shelf-life, it is a pointless exercise that simply leaves food with no nutritional benefit. As food is our main source of nutrition and is essential to help our bodies function, what is the point in eating anything that does not fulfil that purpose? White flour has had 70% of the fiber removed from it and 80% of its vitamins and minerals have been eradicated. This is why you see marketing labels proclaiming their refined products have 'high fiber' and are 'enriched with vitamins and minerals.' Seems silly to eat these versions when you can just opt for whole grains, which have the nutritional benefits that nature intended!

In particular, the fiber found in whole grains is important for our digestive health. Without it, carbohydrates immediately get turned into sugar, which give us short bursts of energy, but leave us feeling hungry and craving more energy only a short time later. Most Americans consume less than 50% of the recommended daily allowance of fiber. This could be a key indicator as to why so many Americans are obese. Also, we know that fiber is a vital ingredient in cleansing our bodies of toxic waste. A lack of fiber can result in a build-up of this waste, commonly known as constipation, which can be painful and result in further complications.

The Glycemic Index (GI) can be useful in helping us decide which carbohydrates are good and which are bad. It indicates how much sugar is readily in food, which then tells us how it will affect our blood sugar level. Higher GI ratings relate to sugar-laden foods, whereas wholegrain foods, fruits, and vegetables rank low on the GI rating. Foods low on the GI are metabolized slower, leaving you feeling fuller for longer, and don't dramatically affect your blood sugar levels. If you are in any doubt about what foods to eat on your journey to improved health, be smart and be sure to check their ranking on the Glycemic Index.

### Is sugar really the enemy?

*Added* sugar is the single worst ingredient in any person's diet. It contributes absolutely NOTHING to your health or wellbeing and has instead been linked to harmful effects on metabolism as well as risks of countless other diseases. Here, we are going to look at some reasons why added sugar should be avoided at all costs!

### 1. Sugar is high in calories and low in, well everything else!

As we have seen, sugar provides a complete calorie-fest without providing you with any nutrition at all in return. Not even one mineral or vitamin! Seems a little one-sided if you ask us! That is why many people refer to sugar as 'empty calories'. If you were to consume more than 20% of your calories as sugar, you would be putting yourself at severe risk of nutrient deficiencies, which in turn have severe effects on your health.

### 2. Sugar wrecks your teeth.

Sugar provides easily digestible energy for the bad bacteria lurking in your mouth to feed off of, putting you at increased risk of cavities and infections in the tooth and gum. Even dentists recommend being cautious of consuming too many natural sugars as they can have a muted version of the same effect.

### 3. Sugar can lead to insulin resistance.

Insulin resistance is one of the stepping stones to Metabolic Syndrome, which we discussed earlier in this chapter. Insulin is a vital hormone that regulates glucose levels by directing our body to burn glucose instead of fat. Too much glucose in the blood stream is toxic and can result in serious complications, such as blindness and amputations. Dozens of studies have linked diets containing large levels of sugar consumption to insulin resistance.

### 4. Insulin resistance, caused by sugar, can lead to diabetes.

If our bodies become resistant to the effects of insulin, our pancreas, which makes it, goes into overdrive to produce enough. The more resistant we become, the harder the pancreas has to work to produce enough insulin to regulate our blood sugar levels until it cannot keep up any longer and our blood sugar levels are so high that Type II diabetes is diagnosed. One study confirms this risk as it found that participants who drank sugar-sweetened drinks had an 83% higher risk of developing diabetes.

## 5. Sugar consumption can overwork your liver.

Fructose is a key component of sugar. Unlike glucose, we cannot produce it ourselves, but we have no need to as it does not benefit us in any way. However, if we consume sugar, we will also consume fructose, which can only be metabolized by the liver. While small amounts can be turned into glycogen and safely stored there for later use, over-consumption of sugar will lead to a build-up of glycogen and the liver will instead be forced to turn the fructose into fat. Fatty livers have been linked to numerous serious health problems including NAFLD – Non Alcoholic Fatty Liver Disease. It is important to add that it is virtually impossible to get too much fructose through fruit consumption and that people who are healthy and active can tolerate more sugar than those who lead a sedentary lifestyle. Consuming more sugar than you can burn is one sure way to get started on creating a fatty liver.

## 6. Sugar is addictive.

Just as is seen in drug and alcohol addicts, sugar causes a release of dopamine in the brain. This is very dangerous for people who are susceptible to addiction as they may find themselves strongly addicted to sugar. For this reason, energy drinks are becoming an increasing addiction for many people who rely on the highs and short bursts of energy they get from drinking it. For example; a 20oz bottle of Mountain Dew energy drink contains a whopping 77 GRAMS of sugar!

## 7. Sugar, not fat, raises your cholesterol.

Historically, saturated fat has been blamed as the primary cause of heart disease. However, more recent studies have begun to show that sugar may be a leading cause of the condition, principally due to the dangerous effects of fructose on our metabolism. Large amounts of fructose can raise triglycerides, LDL, insulin, and blood glucose levels in as little as ten weeks. All of which put you at major risk of heart disease.

## 8. Sugar consumption has been linked to cancer.

Cancer cells are characterized by unregulated multiplication and growth of our body's cells. We have several ways in which our bodies try and regulate this behaviour; including the production of insulin. Some scientists and researchers believe that frequently elevated levels of insulin can contribute to a lack of efficiency in maintaining our cell regulation and, as such, cancer is more of a risk. There are numerous studies that have been done that have concluded that people who eat large amounts of sugar are at a much higher risk of cancer.

## 9. Sugar is a major contributor to obesity.

The two components of sugar: glucose and fructose have slightly different effects on our body. Research was undertaken looking at the ability of sugar-sweetened beverage consumers to feel full after a drink. During the study, the consumers were split into two groups, with one group given a fructose-sweetened drink and the other given a glucose-sweetened drink. The results showed that the group given the fructose-sweetened drink felt hungrier sooner. Other studies have supported this, one showing that fructose was substantially less effective in lowering ghrelin, the hunger hormone, than glucose was.

This section represents a snapshot of some of the studies that have been undertaken into the effects of added sugar. Hopefully, it will highlight how it is detrimental to our health and wellbeing, and why it should be avoided as much as possible.

## Hydrogenated Oils

Hydrogenated oils are vegetable oils with an altered chemical structure designed to increase shelf life and save money for food manufacturers. Hydrogenated oils are also called Trans fats, taking their name from the transformation process that sees unsaturated fat levels decrease and saturated fat levels rise. The process, called hydrogenation, also makes the oil either partially or fully solid when at room temperature. Examples of food products with Trans-fat include: margarine, ready-made cakes and biscuits, and most pastries. One estimate suggests that 40% of food products in the US contain them.

Trans- fat lowers your good cholesterol and raises the bad, making you more at risk of heart disease. Also, they block our natural anti-inflammatory systems, exposing us to inflammation, which has been linked to the development of some cancers. Research by the *Harvard School of Public Health* has reported that Trans- fats over stimulate our immune systems and has links to diabetes, stroke, and other chronic conditions. Another study has suggested that consuming just 5g of Trans- fat per day could increase our risk of heart disease by approximately 25%.

## How can I avoid consuming Trans- fats?

Reading nutrition labels and ingredients lists can be very confusing. Manufacturers have various loopholes that they use to disguise the true components of a product. For example; the FDA guidelines allow manufacturers to use the term 'zero grams Trans-fat' on nutritional information, provided the product contains less than 0.5 grams per serving. Obviously, this is pretty sneaky on their part. It may not contain much, but it still contains some! Your best bet is to check the ingredients list for the words 'partially hydrogenated' or 'hydrogenated'. If these words are present, than so is Trans-fat!

**Alcohol**

Alcohol is the product derived from the fermentation of fruits, cereals, and vegetables. Many health plans completely ban the consumption of alcohol, but it can be included in a healthy lifestyle provided it is enjoyed in moderation. This is why most countries have introduced guidelines as to how much alcohol is considered safe and pose the least risk to your health.

Alcohol contains a toxic chemical called acetaldehyde. If we were to drink too much alcohol on a regular basis for a prolonged period of time, we would be consuming far too much acetaldehyde and be at risk of numerous serious health problems including cirrhosis of the liver.

**How does our body process alcohol?**

The urban legend about drinking on an empty stomach is actually true. We absorb alcohol through our stomach and small intestine, but the rate of absorption is much slower when we have a full belly. This means that the alcohol takes significantly longer for us to 'feel it.' Once it hits our stomach, it is broken down by an enzyme called ADH, which stands for Alcohol Dehydrogenase. Once alcohol is broken down, it journeys through the intestines and to our liver, where it is further deconstructed via a series of molecular transformations. This deconstruction happens in three stages.

1. The alcohol is broken down into toxic acetaldehyde.

2. Then, this is broken down into harmless acetate.

3. Finally, it is reduced to water and carbon dioxide.

Approximately 90-95% of alcohol is broken down by our liver and the remaining percentage excreted through our breath, sweat, and urine. The rate at which this happens will vary dependent on a number of factors including:

gender, age, and weight. The fact that women have different drinking guidelines to men is due to this scientific fact rather than any sexist connotations! The typical rate of absorption is approximately ten grams of alcohol per hour. This is also the reason why many people are found to be over the drink-drive limits the morning after a particularly heavy drinking session. If you were to drink ten cans of beer, you should allow at least ten hours for your body to completely eliminate all of the alcohol you have consumed.

## What are the health risks from drinking more than the recommended guidelines?

Surprisingly, research has demonstrated that those who drink light to moderate amounts of alcohol actually live longer than those who are at either extreme end of the spectrum – that is those people who abstain completely and those who drink excessively. Also, it has a few equally surprising health benefits, specifically helping to lower levels of bad cholesterol and thinning the blood to reduce the risk of stroke, heart attacks, or other thrombosis. One drink will give you the blood-thinning benefit for roughly 24 hours. The key to alcohol is to follow the recommended guidelines. Be aware: there are many medications that strongly discourage the consumption of alcohol while taking them. If you are in any doubt, please check with your doctor or pharmacist.

## Gluten

Gluten and the effects of it on our health has become a very popular topic in recent years and one survey in 2013 identified that one third of Americans were trying to completely eliminate gluten from their diets. Avoiding gluten is seen by many people as a new-age, faddy notion, but there is actually a number of very good reasons to stay away from this protein composite.

We have already briefly explored the problems with refined carbohydrates and the same concerns are echoed in the consumption of gluten. Gluten is found in carbohydrates, like flour, and when mixed with water becomes a sticky, stodgy texture. When the gluten reaches some of our immune system cells located in our gut, our immune system treats it as a foreign enemy and those of us with gluten intolerance will see our immune systems go into overdrive rallying against it. Gluten intolerance, otherwise known as celiac disease, is classified as an autoimmune condition because of the way our bodies react to gluten in our diets.

Overreaction of our immune systems can also cause the intestinal walls to degenerate, not to mention cause other health concerns including: anaemia, irritable bowel syndrome, and many more. Despite all this, up to 80% of adults are unaware that they actually have celiac disease. Even if you do not suffer with full blown celiac disease, many of us still have certain gluten intolerances; causing bloating, severe stomach discomfort, and fatigue. Many of these symptoms are grouped together under the umbrella term, 'Irritable Bowel Syndrome'.

As well as stomach conditions, gluten has also been directly linked to a number of neurological disorders including: cerebellar ataxia, epilepsy, autism, and schizophrenia. Some studies have shown huge improvements in these conditions by eliminating gluten completely from their diets.

During this chapter, we have taken the time to examine the way in which our bodies process certain aspects of our food and drink including calories and alcohol. We have looked into some 'naughty' foods and discovered what they are and what they do to us to enable us to make informed decisions about what we put into our bodies. Continuing this journey in the next chapter, we are going to look at GMO's – Genetically Modified Organisms; what they are, why they exist, and what they mean for us.

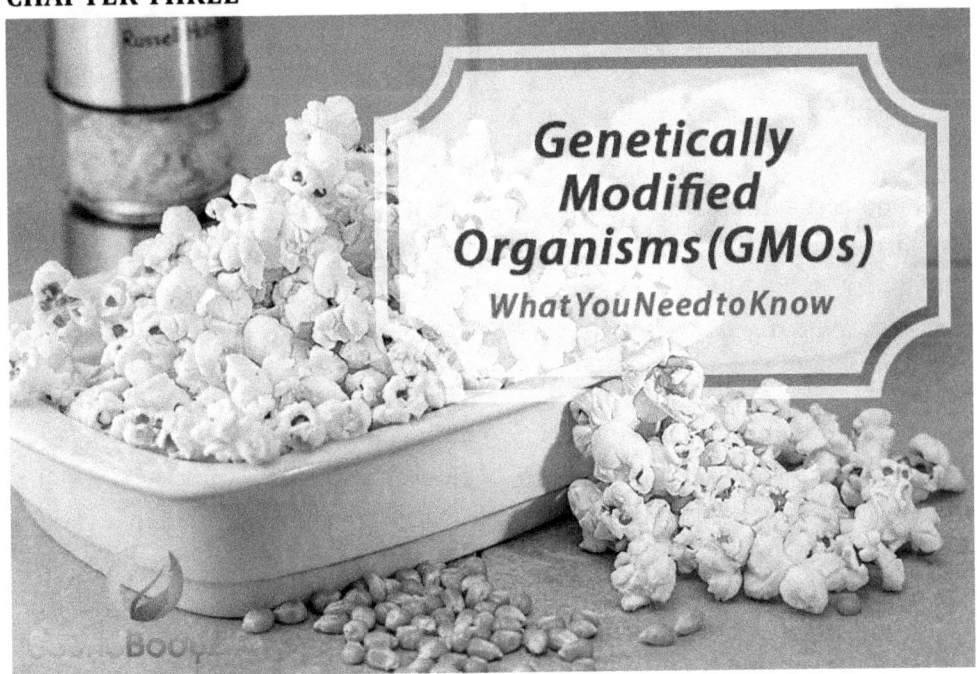

# CHAPTER THREE

## What are GMOs?

GMO stands for *genetically modified organism* – basically living organisms that have had their genetic material artificially manipulated using genetic engineering. The genetic modification involves the insertion, deletion, or mutation of genes. These processes are done in laboratories and result in the creation of unstable combinations of genes from animals, plants, bacteria, and viruses that would not occur either naturally or through normal crossbreeding. GMOs are used in medical and biological research, agriculture, experimental medicine, and the production of pharmaceutical drugs.

## Where are GMOs used?

The first organisms subjected to genetic modification were bacteria, thanks to their simple genetics. They continue to be important in the field of genetic engineering and medicine, with genetically modified bacteria being used to produce human proteins including insulin, vital in the treatment of diabetes. Similar bacteria have been used to create human growth hormones and blood clotting agents, among other medical uses.

GMOs are regularly used as enzymes in the manufacturing of various processed foods. Examples include: Chymosin from fungi or a bacterium which acts as a clotting agent for milk, protein in order to make cheese, and alpha-amylase which converts starch to simple sugars.

Genetic modification has been used in crops in order to provide resistance to pests and herbicides. Other developments include: the production of crops that can thrive within non-native environments or withstand changed conditions within their native environment, for example; a drought or extreme temperature changes. Some plants, including algae and maize, have been modified in order to produce fuel known as bio fuel.

Plants have been subjected to genetic modification in order to produce new wider ranges, including unusual colors of flowers such as the blue rose. GMO's are also utilized in the field of animal research, where they are used in a variety of ways. Not only are they capable of producing new species, as we have seen in their use on plants, but they are also utilized to improve animal health, research human diseases by developing animal models to monitor disease progression, and to enhance food and production traits within the animals themselves.

## Are GMOs safe?

Our primary concern for the focus of this chapter is the consumption of GMO crops and products and what potential effects that this could have on both our immediate and long term health.

There is huge controversy surrounding the use of GMO's in food, with disputes involving scientists, government organisations, government regulators, buyers, and biotechnology businesses. The fundamental issues relate to the labelling of GMO food, the effect of pesticide production and herbicide resistance, the role of government regulators, and the effect of GMO crops both in terms of health and the environment for feeding the world population.

While labelling GMO products are required in some countries, the United States FDA does not necessitate any labelling or distinctions to be made between GMO and non-GMO products. We will look further into labelling and the role of the FDA in a later chapter, but the fact remains that if you are a U.S. citizen, there is no requirement for manufacturers to make you aware that you are consuming genetically modified produce. This makes it extremely difficult for us to make informed food choices for ourselves and our families.

One of the main health concerns surrounding GMO food products relates to the fact that they are engineered to be herbicide tolerant and, as such, GMO crops are subjected to the harsh chemicals used in such herbicides.

## Herbicide Tolerance

Crops that have been genetically modified in order to tolerate broad-spectrum herbicides are very popular with many farmers. This is because they allow for the herbicide to kill the surrounding weeds without affecting the cultivated crop. Currently, the only varieties cultivated in the United States are engineered to be tolerant to the herbicide glyphosate, although the US Department of Agriculture (USDA) is in the process of deregulating other new varieties of crops that have resistance to other herbicides.

Crops that are resistant to glyphosate have been given the term 'roundup ready'. *Roundup* is the name given to a brand of this herbicide that is widely used in everything from large scale agriculture to backyard vegetables patches. It is the number one most commonly used chemical in the U.S. Round-up ready crops, which have dominated United States agriculture in recent years, with a 2010 report from the USDA and NASS (National Agricultural Statistics Service) showing that the use of glyphosate has dramatically increased. Other data illustrates that 57 million pounds of glyphosate was used on U.S corn fields in 2010, compared to only 23 million pounds used in 2005, only five years earlier.

Once applied to crops, the glyphosate transfers the systemic herbicide to the fruit, shoot regions, and roots of the plant. The absorption of the herbicide by the plant means that is cannot be removed from the product by milking, baking or brewing the grains, or by washing or peeling it. Some studies have shown that traces of glyphosate have been evident in food products up to two years later. This means that despite all of our efforts, crops treated with Roundup cannot possibly have all traces of the chemicals removed.

**Surely if the USDA and FDA allow for Roundup to be used on crops, then it is safe for me to consume the chemical residue left on them?**

This is the key question relating to genetically modified produce. While there is broad consensus that food produce derived from GMO crops poses no greater risk than conventional food, the fact remains that by consuming foods that have been treated with herbicides, we are putting unnatural chemicals into our bodies and we have no way of knowing what effect they may be having.

These concerns have been echoed by a number of groups that are opposed to the use of genetically modified foods including: Greenpeace, the Union of Concerned Scientists, and the Organic Consumers Association. They believe that the risks of consuming GMO crops have not been adequately identified or managed and they do not consider the potential long term health impact on human health that GMO crops may have. They support the idea of mandatory labelling, which would allow consumers to be properly informed if the products they are purchasing have derived from GMO food sources.

Although, GMO crops for the agriculture industry may be 'Roundup Ready', we as humans are not. So, we are going to have a look at a few of the documented health concerns relating to the consumption of GMO crops that have been treated with glyphosate and the other 'inactive' chemicals found in Roundup herbicides.

## Negative impact on Stomach Health

Research has shown that glyphosate can cause extreme disruption to the body's internal microflora, actually working to destroy the beneficial bacteria that keeps our gut healthy and balances our other essential bodily mechanisms. The eradication of healthy bacteria allows for toxic pathogens to take over, potentially leading to gastrointestinal conditions, such as inflammatory bowel disease, colitis, and Crohn's disease.

There has also been some evidence linking glyphosates to gluten intolerance as a chemical reaction binding it to the gluten in our stomach, making it highly indigestible. Over time, your body could develop an immune reaction to this chemical reaction, resulting in celiac disease.

## Links to cancer

The International Agency for Research on Cancer (IARC), the principal research arm of the World Health Organization has, in 2015, declared that glyphosate is probably carcinogenic to humans, rating it at 2A on their scale of carcinogenicity. Although several studies have shown an increased risk of non-Hodgkin lymphomas in people who work with the herbicide, other studies have found no links. The Environmental Protection Agency has classified glyphosate as a Group E carcinogen, which means that it has evidence of non-carcinogenicity for humans. However, other evidence from animal research has shown a direct link between glyphosate and tumors found in test-subject rats.

The study, published in *Food and Chemical Toxicology,* showed that exposure over two years to the same genetically modified corn found in the United States food supply resulted in the formation of massive tumors in the animals, some of which weighed in at 25% of their total body weight. The females developed mammary tumors first, followed by pituitary ones. Similar tumors also developed in the male rats. Significant kidney and liver damage was witnessed thanks to changes in the endocrine function and metabolism, including increased ammonia levels in the blood.

So why haven't we seen similar results in humans? Well, the answer may lie in life expectancy. With the average rat living for approximately two to two and a half years, it is reasonable to expect to see results of exposure to GMO crops much sooner in animals than in humans. In the meantime, we are seeing a huge increase in the number of people experiencing chronic diseases, which may represent the early stages of the population battling with the effects of GMO's in their food.

## Links to Alzheimer's disease and Autism

Alzheimer's disease is a severe form of dementia and is reported to be the sixth leading cause of death in the United States. It is driven by poor lifestyle choices and a build-up of toxins in the brain, which is mostly contributed to by poor digestion and stomach health. Our gut directly affects certain hormone levels within the brain including serotonin, which is responsible for much of our behaviour and moods. Serotonin deficiency has been implicated in a host of diseases and conditions including: autism, Alzheimer's, and depression. A characteristic feature of children with autism is an overgrowth of pathogens in the gut, where the toxins produced by these pathogens affect our brain. Various graphic results show a direct correlation between glyphosate usage and autism rates.

A by-product of glyphosate entering our bodies is the production of ammonia. Ammonia is toxic to us and elevated levels of blood ammonia can adversely affect brain function. Research has shown that children with autism tend to have notably higher levels of ammonia in their blood than non-autistic children. Similarly, ammonia is responsible for encephalitis (brain inflammation) seen in patients suffering from Alzheimer's disease.

## Weed Resistance and Herbicides

There is no stopping natural evolution and this is evident with the emergence of herbicide-resistant weeds. The International Survey of Herbicide Resistant Weeds has recorded a massive 522 resistant weeds across the United States. They have evolved in response to the repeated use of herbicides seen in the last few decades. This hasn't happened due to genetic modification of the plants themselves, but because the natural resistance found in a few plants ensured their survival and reproduction. As each generation of the plant becomes more exposed to herbicides, the number of resistant plants increases until they equal and then dominate the susceptible plants.

Studies have shown that farmers who grow genetically modified crops use up to 25% more herbicides than those who grow from regular seeds. With the resistance growing, some farmers have been using even more than normal in the hope that they work, as it is more cost-effective than traditional labor intensive methods of weed removal. Obviously, the more herbicide that farmers use, the greater the number of chemicals absorbed by the plant which are then passed through to us on consumption. This could increase the health risks associated with GMOs by an unprecedented number.

The debate surrounding genetically modified food products and GMOs in general will continue to rage until enough concrete evidence is provided for authorities to realize the risks associated with them. Hopefully, in time, it will be a requirement in every country for GMO warnings to be prevalent on the packaging of products, so that we as consumers can make the food choices that are best for us. However, in the meantime, the risks are clear and evident for all to see. Whether you consider them big enough, is a personal preference, but the fact remains that by consuming genetically modified food, you are opening your body to unnatural chemicals that we simply weren't supposed to consume. The answer to the question of is GMO foods safe is still a ways off, but in the meantime, is it really worth taking the chance that they might be harmful, if not now, then in the future?

In the next chapter, we are going to look further at what we put into our bodies and what the arguments are for going organic. For the meat eaters among us, we are going to explore the importance of knowing where your meat comes from and, most importantly, what the animal ate when it was alive. Also, we are going to touch briefly again on GMOs and the threat of gene transfer from crop to person, and what this could mean for the human population.

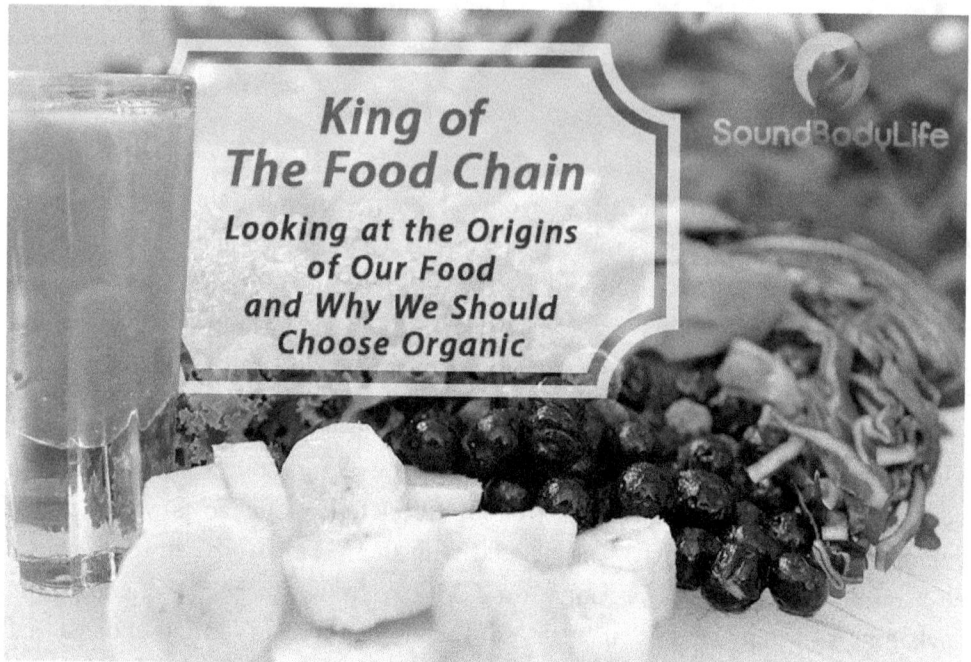

# CHAPTER FOUR

## You are what you eat.

"You are you eat," is a phrase that we have all heard, but this chapter is going to delve into the deepest, darkest depths of our stomachs and examine the importance of knowing what we eat and what we've eaten has eaten! Yes, the food chain is real and it means knowing what goes in at the bottom of it that we can truly make informed food choices. We are also going to look at the reasons why we should be eating organic produce and the effect that antibiotic resistance and gene transfers from genetically modified foods can have on our bodies.

## What does 'eating organic' really mean?

There are many mixed messages about what the term 'organic' really means. In simple terms, if something is organic, then it has been grown without the use of synthetic fertilizers, pesticides, genetically modified organisms, ionizing radiation, or sewage sludge. For an animal to have organic produce, such as dairy products, eggs, or the meat itself, it must not have been given growth hormones or antibiotics.

When it comes to labelling, however, the United States Department of Agriculture (USDA) has three categories and they are as follows:

- 100% Organic
  As expected this means the product is made with 100% organic ingredients.

- Organic
  This label can be applied to products where at least 95% of the ingredients are organic.

- Made with Organic Ingredients
  These products are made with at least 70% organic ingredients, but there are strict regulations and restrictions on the remaining 30%, including prohibiting any GMO's.

  Products that have less than 70% organic ingredients are not able to make any organic claims on the front of their packaging, but they may list organically produced ingredients on the sides of the package.

So, already we can see that the concept of 'organic' may not be as straightforward as we would like to believe.

**Why is organic food so much more expensive?**

One of the arguments that many people have against organic food is the price tag that comes with it, believing that by using the word organic, farmers are just ramping up their profit margins. An actual fact: many organic products do not cost any more than their conventional equivalents, particularly for 'staple' dietary produce like bread, coffee, and cereals. In the last decade, the price of organic food has dropped significantly and experts predict that it will continue to fall as demand grows.

So, why does it appear so expensive? Well, part of the reason is that organic farming is much more expensive than traditional farming. It is substantially more labor intensive and requires significantly more management and organization. Organic farmers also don't receive any federal subsidiaries like conventional farmers. As such, they need to cover the true costs of product growth rather than a subsidized version of it. Finally, organic farms rarely benefit from mass production economies of a scale like traditional farms, due to their smaller size and turnover.

**Animal Products**

It might surprise you to know, but consuming less animal products is actually beneficial to the environment. Animal agriculture produces huge amounts of water and air pollution and it is the cause of 80% of the annual deforestation across the globe. Also, it is a drain on the global grain harvest with 50% being consumed by livestock. Choosing to support local, sustainable, and organic farms is a better choice for you, your family, and your local ecological area. Making informed decisions about the animal products you eat is both your right and your responsibility.

Here are just some of the reasons why you should go organic for your animal products.

## Mad Cow Safeguard

Mad Cow disease, also known as Bovine Spongiform Encephalopathy (BSE), is a fatal neurological condition that affects the central nervous system of adult cattle. Livestock are often fed the ground up remains of other cattle, essentially forcing them into cannibalism. If the deceased animal has died due to BCE, than the remains will likely be infected with the consumption of them responsible for passing the disease on. If humans consume diseased tissue from affected cattle, then they may develop the human equivalent, Creutzfeldt-Jakob disease. Once the infected animal in ingested, the disease has an extended latency period and symptoms may not come to light for several years. When they do, they manifest in a number of ways including: mobility difficulties, depression, and dementia. Brain function and mobility continues to deteriorate and most people with the disease die within a year of the onset of their symptoms due to vulnerability to infection. If you opt to purchase organic meat, you can be certain that the animal which you are eating has not been fed anything other than 100% organic feed.

## Better treatment of animals

Organic animal produce tends to be packaged with the terms 'free range' or 'ranch raised'. These indicate that the animals were raised in a much better, more humane way. They are less restricted in terms of movement and most spend plenty of time outdoors rather than cooped up in cages. They also normally have a better diet, which they are allowed to eat when they need to, rather than at prescribed times with specified amounts. There have been a number of studies that suggest that animals raised in this way produce better quality food items.

## Manure

Manure is a natural soil fertilizer and is used on farms for this purpose. Industrial farms produce huge amounts of waste, for example; hog farms in North Carolina produce approximately 10 million metric tons of waste per year. This manure can become filled with E.coli and other pathogens, causing an extreme health risk, particularly if there is no regulation as to what diet is fed to their animals. Smaller sustainable farms that feed their animals exclusively organic feed can be sure that their manure is also organic. Therefore, it can be utilized effectively and safely as a fertilizer on their farms.

## Fewer chemicals used

Organic farms do not allow the use of synthetic pesticides or fertilizers on either the food or their land. Instead, they prefer to use traditional farming methods, such as crop rotation, to improve soil fertility and increase productivity. They also refuse to feed their animals any food that contains pesticides. Therefore, these chemicals cannot be passed through to the consumer. Organic farming focuses on what nature provides rather than relying on chemical ways to control the environment. This affects not only the products that you buy, but it also safeguards the groundwater, the local habitat, and the health of the farmers.

## It's good to be green!

The majority of factory farms are run with non-renewable fossil fuels and without this, the process of creating, producing, transporting, and marketing the foods would be impossible. However, it is very costly to the environment. Supporting local organic farms is a better choice. Not only do they use 70% less energy than industrial farms, which is environmentally friendly, but your food will have less distance to travel; meaning that it will arrive to you fresher and tastier than before!

## Free of... well everything!

Animals that are raised as organic are not allowed to be subjected to artificial interference from antibiotics, hormones, or any other drugs. They are forbidden from eating GMO food products and cannot have their own genes modified. Organically raised animals have been demonstrated to be comparably healthier than those which have been raised in factories under confinement. Updates and further information on U.S. federal organic standards can be found on the Organic Trade Association website.

## Support your local businesses.

Why put your hard earned money into big business corporations by buying non-organic, mass produced produce when you could be supporting your local farms directly. By purchasing straight from nearby organic farms, you can guarantee that your dollars are going to go straight back into their business, helping them to continue to provide you and your local community with healthy organic produce for years to come.

## We are what they eat?

As humans, we are at the top of the food chain. While we may think this puts us in a position of strength, it actually makes us vulnerable to bacteria, pathogens, drugs, contaminants, and anything else that could be lurking in the food of the animals that we consume. Before GMO feed was created, animals used to eat whatever grew naturally for them. Chickens and cows would eat grass and grains, and bigger fish would eat smaller sea life. However, the sheer size of industrial farms, some with 30,000 cows or 60,000 chickens, has meant that it is virtually impossible to feed them in this way. Sadly, the need for safe ways to dispose of slaughtered animals and the requirement for huge rations of protein-rich food paved the way for a mutual agreement between farmers and slaughterhouses to include animal by-products (ground up carcasses) in animal feed. Nice huh?

While this process has solved their immediate concerns with regards to providing food and dealing with waste, it has created a whole host of issues in terms of controlling, monitoring, and regulating the practice. It has also led to countless health concerns including those surrounding BSE (mad cow disease).

## The 1997 Feed Ban

In 1997, the United States Food and Drug Administration (FDA) declared that protein from cud-chewing animals should be kept out of animal feeds in an attempt to keep the supply free from infectious prions, which were the proteins that they believed caused BSE. While the rendering process eliminated most harmful viruses and bacteria, it did not destroy all of the offending prions. The ban was orchestrated to prevent cattle from consuming infected feed, thus reducing the possibility of it being passed to humans, where it could cause fatal brain disease. However, loopholes were found, enforcement was lax, and industry compliance with the ban has been flawed. Between 2007 and 2013, 47 different companies recalled more than 280 feed products that were in violation of the federal rules.

So what is the FDA doing now? According to their website, since 2009 they have made additional effort to ensure food safety, stating that certain high-risk cow parts are forbidden from being used to make any animal feed, including that for pets. The parts that are considered to be high-risk are those parts of the animal that have the highest chance of being affected by the infected prion, including the brain and spinal cord from cows beyond 30 months of age. The FDA has also stated that they are working in conjunction with the USDA to prevent high-risk cattle from entering the United States and ensuring that the high risk parts of the cow that are removed are properly disposed of. At the current time, the last cow recorded with BSE in the United States was in 2012.

It would appear that the regulatory agencies are making effort to provide preventative measures to reduce the chance of contaminated meat getting into our food supply. Despite their efforts, there is still some risk. Can they truly guarantee that there is no way the supply could become infected? Surely it would be better to do away with this method of feeding cattle altogether? The only way we can guarantee that our meat is free from BSE is to ensure that we buy organic.

**So what exactly do they eat?**

In order to know exactly what we are putting into our bodies, we need to begin at the bottom of the food chain with what our food sources put into theirs.

Non-organic chickens and cattle are given primarily plant-based feed, a mixture of corn and soy bean. This accounts for between 70 and 90 percent of most commercial animal feeds. However, the remaining percentage of their food can vary hugely from what they would eat in their natural habitat. Examples of what makes up the rest of the percentage can include: plastic pellets, floor waste from chicken coops including faecal matter, and processed feathers. In industrial farming, the motto is to fatten up their animals as quickly and cheaply as possible in order to make the biggest profits.

Also included in the feed can be an array of medication that is given to cattle and poultry regardless of whether they need it, which encourages growth and helps prevent infection and illness. There is no way of knowing exactly how much of what animals consume actually passes through to us.

More recently, there has been disturbing reports of farmers reverting to feeding their animals discarded junk food. Yes, really. Foods such as French fries, candy bars, chips, and cookies have been replacing corn-based feeds. The reason for this, as you can probably expect, comes back to cost. The price of corn has more than doubled and it is becoming more cost effective for farmers to feed their stock diets of discarded junk food than purchase commercial feeds.

## GMO feed vs. non-GMO feed

An increasing number of farmers have been reporting health problems with animals that have been fed genetically modified feed and noticing a substantial improvement in their wellbeing when switching to non-GMO alternatives. Agriculture advisors have stated that animals have gained weight faster and had better overall reproduction and health when fed non-GMO feed. A study of pigs consuming GMO feed in actual farm conditions, published in 2013, found that the animals suffered with severe stomach inflammation. The number of pigs affected was significantly higher than results found in pigs that were fed non-GMO feed. Other health problems resulting from GMO feeds which have been noted include; botulism in dairy cows, reproductive difficulties and viral diseases in beef cows and hogs, and rickets and bowel issues in hogs. These health concerns have been especially prevalent in genetically modified corn that has been treated with the herbicide Glyphosate (Roundup).

## Animal Opinion

What if cattle and poultry had their own opinions about which feeds they preferred? There are plenty of farmers who tell stories that suggest that their animals instinctively shun eating GMOs. There are also a number who have reported a reduction in feed use since swapping to non-GMO feeds, citing that livestock needs to eat less in order to be full.

## Genetic Transfer and Antibiotic Resistance

There is evidence that points to the possibility that genetically modified genes in crops of food can transfer from one species to another and potentially cause mutations in bacteria in the new host.

The original study was carried out at the University of Jena and discovered that genes used to modify oilseed rape were transferred to bacteria found in the guts of bees. The oilseed rape was genetically modified to resist a specific strain of herbicide. Oilseed rape pollen was then extracted from the legs of honey bees and fed to immature bees. When the intestines of the immature bees were examined, it was found that some of them carried the gene that was resistant to the herbicide.

So, what implications does potential gene transfer have for us? Well, one of the genes used by agricultural-science companies in their genetic engineering is actually an antibiotic resistant gene. It is applied to genetically modified mixes to help biotechnologists identify which cells have successfully had the foreign DNA transplanted into them. The successful cells will survive, while the unsuccessful ones will die once the antibiotics have been administered.

So what if, like in the study with the bees, antibiotic resistance is passed down to humans who eat the products? A genetics professor at the University in West Ontario, Canada, has stated that many of the antibiotics used in surgery and the treatment of infections and diseases is the same as that used in GMO crops. If gene transfer were to occur, it could have potentially fatal consequences for us, particularly if we already have low or compromised immune systems.

A British study at the University of Newcastle found that three of seven subjects who ate one meal containing genetically modified soy had traces of the modified DNA found in bacteria in their small intestines. This evidence directly contradicts claims by the GMO industry that the likelihood of genetic transfer from food to human is very small. The British Food Standards Agency (FSA) has downplayed the study, citing that GMO foods are safe and there is no risk to human health. However, the question has been asked if genetically modified DNA was already present in the guts of those individuals? If it wasn't, then this study proves that gene transfer may in fact be quite likely after all.

If the GMO DNA was already present in the bodies of those people, how did it get there? Either it had got into the gut a long time ago and was passed down or people are eating genetically modified soy on a regular basis. Whatever the answer is, the simple fact is: this study proves that if, as the government agencies state, transfer *isn't* possible then there is every chance that millions of people could already have GMO DNA already present inside them.

### Seafood – wild vs farmed: Which is more beneficial?

Approximately 80% of the seafood sold in the United States is imported and the FDA is responsible for ensuring it is safe for consumption. Unfortunately, other countries are less strict when it comes to seafood safety protocol, meaning that there are definite hazards associated with imported seafood.

The same food chain that we have discussed with regards to livestock is also present in marine life. At the top are the predators and much bigger fish that eat the smaller fish. These smaller fish will have eaten even tinier marine life including shrimps, plankton, etc. So once again, in order to know exactly what we are putting into our bodies when we eat fish, we need to start by looking at what goes in at the very bottom of the food chain.

Farmed fish and wild fish can have quite different diets, which is reminiscent of what we have explored in looking at farm animals. To give you one example, we will have a quick look at salmon, which is one of the biggest imported fish in the United States. Salmon is generally considered hugely beneficial to human health, as it has a lot of Omega-3 fatty acids. Omega-3s are beneficial to our hearts and brains. However, the fat in salmon also has a tendency to stockpile toxins that the fish has consumed.

Obviously, in the wild, the salmon only have the option of consuming smaller fish. However, farmed fish are usually fed a mixture of concentrated fish meal and fish oil. A study undertaken at Indiana University and published in a 2004 issue of *Science* found that farmed salmon had greater amounts of PCBs (polychlorinated biphenyls – industrial chemicals) and dioxins that were likely carcinogenic. While each component alone was lower than the FDA's tolerance level, in those fish that had combined concentrations, the levels were high enough to trigger local consumption advisories. The study also found that fish from North and South America were much less contaminated than those imported from Europe.

Although some major international fish feed producers do test their products for contaminants, the FDA has expressed concern that other, smaller producers have included unapproved drugs in their feed mixes, which could potentially pose risks to human health. The other concern is that farmed fish are increasingly being switched to feeds based on vegetable matter. These feeds may result in an accumulation of pesticides within them that can be passed through to us. Our previous chapter, looking at glyphosate and the effects of herbicides on our bodies, will have given you more information on what risks to our health are posed by these potent chemical combinations. While there is inconclusive evidence with regards to the levels of toxicity that humans may be exposed to, there is no doubt that there is still a very real possibility that they could enter our bodies via the fish that we eat.

During this chapter, we have covered a lot of technical information, but we have tried to make it as easy as possible to understand as we believe that a fundamental aspect of switching to a healthy lifestyle is being able to make informed decisions about the food that you eat. We have examined the benefits of organic farming, not just for the consumer, but also for the livestock involved in the process. Also, we have looked at how organic farming is better both for the environment and the local community.

An integral part of eating organic foods means understanding the differences in how livestock on organic farms are raised compared to those on huge industrial units. We have explored the variations in genetically modified and non-genetically modified feed and what this means for the animals and for us as the end consumer. We have taken a glimpse at the risks of gene transfer, antibiotic resistance, and discussed how seafood may be affected in the same way as livestock.

What we have been able to surmise from this chapter is that the very best way to be healthy is to have as much control as possible over what we put into our bodies. By adopting an organic lifestyle, we can greatly limit the number of chemicals, toxins, and other unnatural products that we ingest, potentially saving ourselves from a number of risks that, at the current time, have not been fully or accurately examined.

In the next chapter, we are going to be considering various food and drink regulations, the involvement of the FDA and similar bodies, and whether or not we think they are doing enough. We will explore the influence of big chemical and agricultural businesses on the standards imposed by such agencies. There is a lot of debate surrounding aspartame and we also plan to dispel some of the myths, giving you the information you need to know about this dangerous chemical.

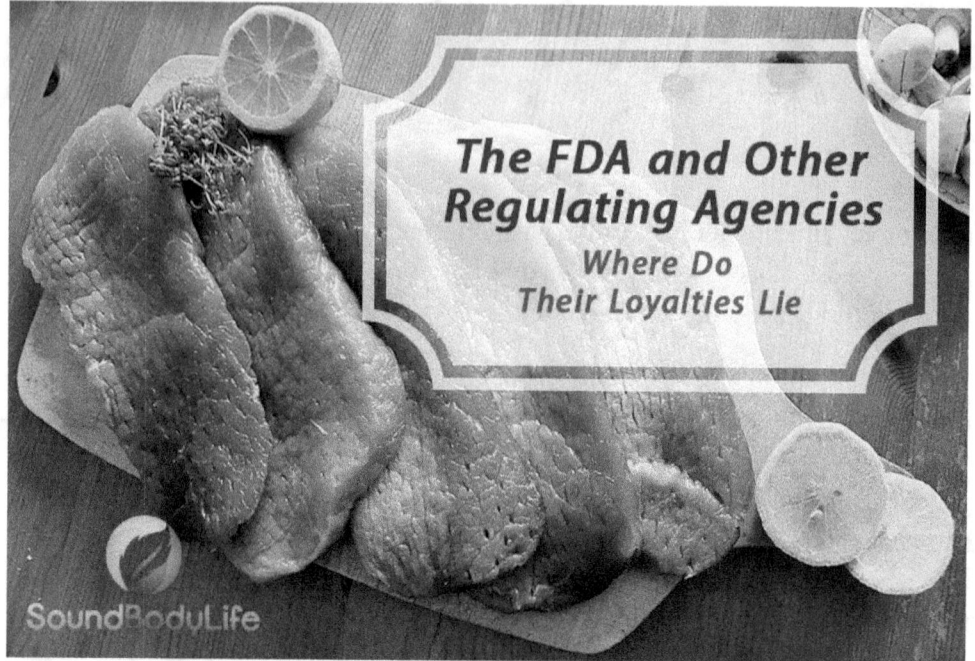

# CHAPTER FIVE

The FDA and Other Regulating Agencies
*Where Do Their Loyalties Lie*

SoundBodyLife

In this chapter, we are going to take a brief look at the United States Food and Drug Administration (FDA) and their role in regulating the food and pharmaceutical industries to ensure our welfare. We are also going to explore the influence that large chemical and agricultural businesses have on the decisions made and standards imposed by the agencies, like the FDA, that are responsible for ensuring the safety of these products. We plan to discuss one of the most controversial, yet legal, substances currently available: Aspartame, and are going to tell you in no uncertain terms what the truth really is about what has been dubbed, 'the most dangerous substance on the market.'

## The FDA

The FDA is the agency that is relied upon by Americans to properly regulate all food and pharmaceutical items, including cosmetics and both human and veterinary drugs. They do this by ensuring the safety, security, and efficiency of these products through rigorous research and testing.

They are also responsible for the advancement of public health by helping to speed up innovations that make drugs affordable, safer, and more effective. They must ensure that the public receives scientifically-based, reliable information to allow them to make informed decisions about how foods and medicines may affect their overall health.

**What exactly does the FDA regulate?**

- Foods, including but not limited to:
    - Food additives
    - Bottled water
    - Dietary supplements
    - Infant formulas
    - Other food products, in conjunction with the U.S. Dept of Agriculture which has a lead role in the regulation of farmed produce
- Drugs:
    - Non-prescription drugs (over the counter)
    - Prescription-only drugs (generic and brand name varieties)

- Biologics, including but not limited to:
    - Allergenics
    - Tissue and tissue products
    - Cellular and gene therapy products
    - Blood and blood products
    - Vaccines

- Medical Devices, including but not limited to:
    - Dental devices
    - Simple medical items, such as tongue depressors
    - Complicated medical items, such as hearing aids
    - Surgical implants and prosthetics

- Cosmetics, including but not limited to:
    - Nail polish and perfumes
    - Skin moisturizers and cleansers
    - Color additives found in make-up and other personal care products

- Electronic Products that emit radiation, including:
    - X-ray equipment
    - Microwave ovens

- Ultrasonic therapy equipment
- Laser products
- Sunlamps
- Mercury vapor lamps

- Veterinary products, including but not limited to:
  - Veterinary drugs and devices
  - Pet foods
  - Livestock feeds

- Tobacco products:
  - Cigarettes
  - Cigarette tobacco
  - Roll-your-own tobacco
  - Smokeless tobacco

Despite their responsibilities, the FDA have come under fire for a large variety of reasons, some of which we will share with you now.

## 1. Poor labelling

In 2009, the FDA came under attack when two safety experts blasted them for leaving important drug information off when listing ingredients on labels. This error was not even highlighted to doctors, who remained unaware about certain drug information, which could have led to catastrophic consequences.

## 2. Lax drug approval

The FDA is only supposed to approve drugs that are safe *and* work effectively, but they work to the rule that approval is granted if the benefits outweigh the side effects. However, this does not guarantee that the drug is either high quality or particularly useful in treating the condition for which it is licensed.

## 3. Tomato-gate

The FDA was to blame for the massive hit that some agriculture companies took in recent years. During one of several cases of a Salmonella outbreak, the FDA assigned blame to tomatoes and people began to avoid eating them, causing huge waste and financial implications for farmers. Florida alone lost most of its harvest thanks to the FDA's error. It was later established that tomatoes had nothing to do with the outbreak.

## 4. Sitting on the fence over questionable data

An article published in the New York Times in 2009 revealed that the FDA often 'sits on' controversial data surrounding the therapeutic or safety values of a drug. Examples include: an antidepressant that demonstrated a side effect of suicidal thoughts and behavior witnessed in children that were taking it. The FDA illustrated a real reluctance to provide an open and transparent service when it came to data analysis.

## 5. Irresponsible approval of drugs

The diabetes drug Avandia has been suspected of killing around 80,000 people, and yet it is still on the market. When questioned regarding its use, the FDA decided that although they knew it was dangerous, clearer warning labels on them would be a sufficient solution.

## 6. They are reluctant to pursue criminal prosecutions

The FDA was pressured by congress to significantly improve its criminal prosecutions of those food and drug companies that failed to meet the stringent criteria imposed, after critics warned that the FDA had failed to maintain high developing performance standards.

## 7. Stock scandals

A chemist within the FDA, along with his son, was charged with amassing a $3.6 million fortune through insider trading after using classified information about drug approvals to make beneficial trades.

## 8. Failure to comment on a test subject's suicide

During testing of a new antidepressant drug, a 19 year old test subject committed suicide by hanging in the laboratory of an Indianapolis-area drug company. Since no negative side effects had been shared by the manufacturer with regards to the drug she was taking, the FDA was expected to share and continue their research in an effort to understand why the suicide took place. However, they refused to comment, citing it would not be in the drug company's best interests.

## 9. The FDA leaders are in the pockets of drug company bosses

A number of FDA scientists have rallied against their own agency for favoring the wishes of drug companies over scientific evidence. President Obama received a letter from one such group of worried scientists who believed that their leaders were corrupt and in the pocket of drug company bosses. The scientists also accused their leaders of violating their own laws by altering scientific findings, making false statements in official FDA documents, removing black box warnings, and approving a mammogram device after it was unanimously vetoed by FDA experts.

## 10. Most American's believe the FDA is not impartial

Surveys have shown that four out of five Americans think that the FDA is heavily influenced by its relationship with drug companies and 96% would like the government to ensure that warning labels are placed on drugs with known safety issues.

## 11. How drug decisions are made

Whether approval is given to a drug is decided by a comparison based on deadliness rather than safety. If that drug is no more deadly than any other comparable drug already on the market than it can be approved.

## 12. The FDA were partially responsible for the Vioxx deaths

Vioxx was a popular NSAID pain reliever before studies revealed it caused severe health problems including strokes, heart attacks, and even death among large numbers of Americans. The FDA, along with the drug's manufacturer Merck, was accused of concealing the risks associated with it and refusing to recall it. Claims were also made that the FDA dragged their heels in performing additional clinical trials after concerns were raised and they approved the drug anyway without any recalls or further research.

**So, are the FDA and drug and food manufacturers really partners in crime?**

There are dozens of reports online that show considerable lapses of judgement from the FDA where drug and food manufacturers are concerned. While we could share every single one with you and bombard you with a lot of complicated and detailed information, instead we are going to focus on just one, which should be sufficiently enlightening, to allow you to form your own opinions regarding the relationship between the FDA and manufacturers.

Before the FDA approves drugs for the market, the manufacturers must put them through numerous clinical trials and document the results. However, these results are rarely published by the drug companies and there is currently no legislation in place to make it mandatory to do so, either upon its release into the market or even years down the line. So, why don't the manufacturers share their findings if they have nothing to hide? Instead, they either fail to disclose all of the results of their tests in order to push their drugs through approval at the FDA or the FDA is approving them regardless. Either way, dangerous and potentially fatal drugs are slipping through the cracks and getting onto the market, which is certainly the case for the drug that we are going to examine for this case study, Pradaxa.

# The FDA and Pradaxa

Pradaxa is a prescription blood thinner medication that has been approved by the FDA as a viable alternative to Warfarin. However, substantial safety concerns have been noted regarding its use and increasing number of lawsuits have been filed against the company which manufactures it. According to the clinical trials, it is safer and more effective than Warfarin and the initial safety report released by the FDA stated that the bleeding rates on Pradaxa did not appear to be any higher than that of Warfarin.

So, let's compare the two. Warfarin's side effects make it one of the primary causes of emergency room deaths and, in 2011 alone, it caused 1,106 serious complications and 72 deaths.

However, in 2011, Pradaxa side effects caused 3,781 serious complications, of which 2,367 were haemorrhages. There were also 542 deaths. These statistics represented the highest level of adverse effects in any of the 800 monitored pharmaceutical drugs.

So, once there was clinical proof of the dangers of Pradaxa, surely the most obvious and moral thing to do would be to remove it from sale immediately, right? Not if you are the FDA. While they updated their safety report to reflect that the risk of major bleeding from Pradaxa is six times higher than Warfarin, the FDA still allows for the continued use of the drug. Why you ask? Well, as usual, it all comes back to money. Pradaxa is 60 times more expensive than Warfarin to buy and adds an estimated $1 billion per year to the already bulging pockets of the manufacturers. So take a guess to which blood thinner they would prefer to be selling?

While some of the FDA is funded by the taxpayers, the majority of their budget comes from industry user fees which, you guessed it, are paid by the manufacturers. The FDA budget increase of 2014 reportedly consisted of 770 million dollars—or around 94% of drug companies' money—undoubtedly giving them major leverage over the agency.

Even though there are plenty of safety warnings plastered over the websites and labelling for Pradaxa, the fact that it is clinically proven to be more dangerous than Warfarin means that the FDA are violating their own code of ethics with regards to approval. It is clearly more deadly than the alternative already on the market and, as such, it should be removed from sale immediately.

We hope that this case study gives you an insight into the relationship between the FDA and drug companies, and the credible threat that it poses to the very processes that are supposed to keep us safe.

## Aspartame – not so sweet?

Aspartame is a low-calorie artificial sweetener that is most prevalent in diet versions of popular soft drink brands, including Coca Cola and Pepsi. There has been a lot of controversy surrounding whether it's safe for consumption, as it has been linked to a number of serious health problems, including cancer. We are going to take an in-depth look at what aspartame really is and what effects it can have on your body.

## So what exactly is it?

Aspartame is a compound that is made up of three different components: aspartic acid, methanol, and phenylalanine, which are free-form amino acids. Now, we are going to look at each of these components in turn.

## Aspartic acid

The aspartic acid that is present in aspartame acts as an excitotoxin, which does what it suggests and excites, or over-stimulates, the nerve cells of the body. This effect is not limited to the peripheral nerves but also affects the brain thanks to its free-form state. Excitotoxins have been shown to play a key part in degenerative nervous system diseases; such as Alzheimer's, Parkinson's, and Huntingdon's diseases. Imbalances of excitotoxins have also been shown to affect the 'hardwiring' of the brain by creating abnormal brain pathways. This can result in the development of serious behavioral disorders including: learning disorders, ADD, hyperactivity, and aggression to name just a few. It can also affect the endocrine system, leaving you with health problems, such as infertility, premature puberty, and premature menopause.

## Methanol

Methanol is a poisonous, colorless, and highly flammable liquid which is most often used to make formaldehyde, paint strippers, acetic acid, and methyl t-butyl, which is a gasoline additive. It is also the alcohol most often linked to blindness. It can invade our bodies through our skin and inhalation, as well as by ingesting it. Consumed in Aspartame, the breakdown components of methanol, formaldehyde (a known carcinogen), and formic acid can poison you individually as much as they can when combined together. The methanol is absorbed quickly through the stomach and small intestine, where it is converted to formaldehyde. This is, in turn, converted to formic acid using our own enzymes, leaving us with two highly toxic and cumulative substances in our bodies. These toxins can have very damaging effects on our health, particularly when they are combined with the excitotoxins found in aspartic acid.

## Phenylalanine

Phenylalanine makes up 50% of aspartame and is also an amino acid. However, unlike naturally found amino acids, which are always found in pairs, Phenylalanine has been isolated from it partner, which is only ever done in highly processed products. It is also an excitotoxin, over-stimulating nerves throughout the body and in the brain, and carries the same risks of behavioral conditions and degenerative disease. Phenylalanine is especially dangerous if you are someone who carries the PKU gene, as it can cause irreversible brain damage and even death, particularly during pregnancy or if consumed in very high doses.

What is evident from all three of these components is that each of them contains excitotoxins, which stimulate our neuron receptors, aka our brain cells, at an exponential rate. They fire impulses so quickly that they risk becoming exhausted and 'frying' some cells altogether. Combining multiple excitotoxins together can only escalate this process, substantially increasing all of the subsequent risks associated with them.

## Aspartame Side Effects

So, we have seen that the components of aspartame can potentially have a dangerous effect on our health, but 'over-stimulated neurons' could still be a bit of a vague description. So let's dumb it down a little, what physical effects are we risking by consumption of this substance that is 200 times sweeter than sucrose?

There have been more than 92 different health-related side effects reported that have been associated with the consumption of aspartame. Part of this is due to the fact that aspartame dissolves and journeys around the body via the blood stream. What side effects you may experience is very much dependant on your own genetic makeup and any physical weaknesses you may have. Similarly, adverse reactions may be instant and acute or they may seem to be non-existent, yet are accumulating into long-term damage.

Reported aspartame side effects include:

**Eye Health**

Blindness in one or both eyes

Vision disruption i.e. tunnel vision, blurring, flashes

Degeneration in night vision

Pain in one or both eyes

Problems with tear ducts

Struggles with wearing contact lenses

Inflammation/bulging eyes

**Ear Health**

Substantial hearing impairments

Severe intolerance of noise

Tinnitus

**Neurological Health**

Headaches or migraines

Epileptic seizures

Confusion and/or memory loss

Dizziness and/or loss of balance

Fatigue, drowsiness or sleepiness

Slurring of speech

Paraesthesia or numb limbs

Severe tremors

Unusual face pain

Hyperactivity

Restless legs

**Psychiatric/psychological Health**

Anxiety

Aggression

Irritability

Severe depression

Insomnia

Phobias

Unusual changes in personality

**Chest Health**

Shortness of breath and/or tight chest

Palpitations / tachycardia

Recent spikes in blood pressure

**Gastrointestinal Health**

Pain when swallowing

Nausea

Diarrhea – sometimes blood is present in stools

Abdominal pain

**Skin Health & Allergies**

Aggravation of allergic conditions i.e. asthma

Hives

Swellings

Lip and mouth reactions

Itching without a visible rash

**Metabolic and Endocrine Health**

Hypoglycaemia (low blood sugar)

Menstrual changes

Severe PMS

Struggling to control diagnosed diabetes

Hair thinning or hair loss

Substantial weight loss

Gradual weight gain

**Other Health**

Substantial increased susceptibility to infections

Burning during urination

Excessive thirst

Fluid retention, leg swelling, bloating

**Additional symptoms of aspartame toxicity include:**

Suicidal tendencies

Aggressive behavior

Severe depression

Hyperactivity, particularly in children

Sugar cravings and aspartame addiction

Peptic ulcers

Birth defects

Irreversible brain damage

Death

**Aspartame may trigger, mimic or cause the following illnesses:**

Attention Deficit Disorder (ADD)

Lymphoma

Non-Hodgkin's

Lupus

Fibromyalgia

Mercury sensitivity from Amalgam fillings

Hypothyroidism

EMS

Multiple Sclerosis

Epilepsy

ALS

Alzheimer's disease

Meniere's disease

Grave's Disease

Lyme Disease

Post-Polio Syndrome

Epstein-Barr

Chronic Fatigue Syndrome

(Source: http://www.sweetpoison.com/aspartame-side-effects.html )

## So what does the FDA say about Aspartame?

The subject of aspartame has been a thorn in the side of the FDA since its initial approval in 1974 when they gave it the nod for limited use. This decision was based on the results of safety tests that they had been given by the manufacturers, Searle. Some serious side effects then came to light and the FDA ordered a task force to review the original safety research conducted. The task force discovered that any negative data had been strategically omitted from the reports that had been supplied to the FDA.

Examples of this negative data included that Searle researchers had failed to report all of the tumors removed from animals which had been fed aspartame. They also failed to check these tumors for signs of cancer. Searle was found to have falsified blood test results, apparently due to 'instrument problems'.

When aspartame came up for approval again in 1980, the FDA recommended that a public enquiry be undertaken in order to determine its safety. The three scientists that made up the board for the enquiry made a recommendation that aspartame should be withdrawn from the market until such a time that testing on animals could prove that it did not cause tumors. Not completely satisfied, the results of the public enquiry then went to a Commissioner's team of scientists, but despite a deadlock in the results, the FDA Commissioner at the time, Dr. Goyan, opted not to approve aspartame.

In April 1981, Dr. Arthur Hayes took over as Commissioner and Searle applied for approval once again. Within a few months, Dr. Hayes had approved aspartame for use in dry foods and, in 1983, he granted approval for it to be used in diet soft drinks. Only one month later, Dr. Hayes left the FDA and within three months had a role within Searle's advertising agency, Burson-Marsteller. We will leave it to you to decide if you think this is a coincidence or a strategically planned maneuver?

Regardless of the FDA's decision to approve aspartame, there is significant evidence that there are real dangers associated with the consumption of it and that is the bitter truth.

Aspartame's inconsistent history raises red flags with the FDA's practices as well as with the product itself, which brings us to the conclusion of this chapter. The FDA is supposed to provide an impartial verification of the safety of the products brought to its table for approval, but how can we trust them when we see the failings that we have explored within this chapter.

We know that manufacturers are willing to disregard their moral compass in favor of dollar signs, omitting research and submitting falsified documents in order to push their products through the approval process. Combine this with stories, such as that of Dr. Hayes' sudden career change, and it becomes easy to believe that the FDA is firmly sitting in the pockets of drug companies and food manufacturers. Can we really put our health in their hands?

We hope that this chapter has given you some insight into the role and responsibilities of the FDA, and the processes that they use to decide whether a product passes for approval. We also hope that we have given you enough information about aspartame to allow you make informed choices about the consumption of aspartame.

So, we have given you plenty of information and now to the fun stuff.... really embarking on your new healthy and natural lifestyle! In the next chapter, we are going to help you get started with plenty of advice, suggestions, and tips. Ready? Let's go!

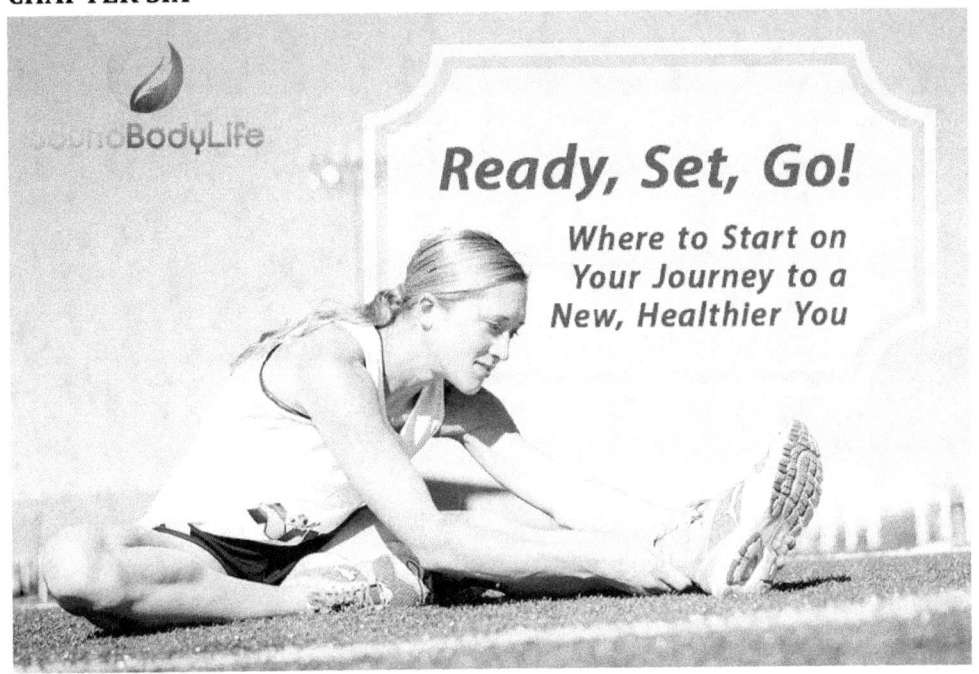

# CHAPTER SIX

*"It's not that some people have willpower and some don't. It's that some people are ready to change and others are not."*

One of the key parts of embarking on a healthy and natural lifestyle is making informed decisions about the process and hopefully the information that we have given you in earlier chapters has made you feel a lot more confident about why you have made this decision. Believe us, this is absolutely the best thing that you could be doing for your overall wellbeing.

The first thing that we are going to look at is your motivation for making the change. Every motivation has its own challenges that relate to it and we are going to help you identify and deal with those hurdles so that you can overcome them on your journey to a new, healthier you.

## Motivations for making the change

*Physical Motivation: "Forget about getting skinny. Eat well and exercise and the weight will take care of itself".*

This quote is awesome, mostly because it is true. A large majority of people who decide to make the change to a healthy lifestyle do so primarily because they do not like what they see when the look in the mirror. We stand in front of the mirror poking at bits of our body we dislike or go into a changing room to try something on and realized the size we have picked up is far too small. Yes, aesthetics is a huge motivation to diet for many people, but it is rarely enough to sustain the transition to regularly picking good choices over bad.

Why isn't it? Well because, for most of us, the battle to change our physical appearance takes too long and we become unmotivated. Let's look at this as if it were a boxing match.

In the red corner, we see ourselves and feel our disgust at our reflection.

In the blue corner, is our food demons, the ones we know will ultimately cause us to put on more weight and worsen how we feel about the way we look.

## Round One

We go into round one feeling energized and motivated. It's hard because we lack physical fitness and we are fighting the cravings, but ultimately we have the upper hand.

## Round Two

The food demons are back for more, but we are ready for them. Again, it's hard going, but our dislike for our physical selves pushes us forward to dominate the fight.

### *Now fast forward to Round Eight*

Round eight starts and we are getting tired. We aren't seeing physical changes quick enough, but we are still fighting just as hard to battle the food demons. They are starting to gain control of the fight.

### *Finally in Round Twelve*

We can't face it anymore. We are sick of fighting the same battle over and over again with little reward. We decide that it isn't worth the effort. We are no skinnier and the food demons are still raging. We give up and the food demons win.

This is exactly what we DON'T want to happen!

So why does it?

- It happens because we set ourselves a goal that is so far in the future it seems impossible.
- It happens because we expect too much from ourselves too quickly.
- It happens because we are impatient. We want to be slim and we want it now.
- It happens because we don't have the tools in place to help us fight our food demons effectively. We don't have to battle them head on. We can be sneaky and Chapter 7 will tell you a lot more about how to do this!

This is not to say that you cannot use aesthetics for some motivation, only that it shouldn't be your only goal, because the most important changes are happening on the inside!

So, in terms of your physical appearance, what can you do to help stay on track? One of the best pieces of advice we can give you is not to weigh or measure yourself too regularly. Sure, this is one of the easiest ways to tell if you are losing weight, but it is also one of the biggest downfalls of motivation if we don't see the results that we are hoping for. All too often, people stand on the scales after a full week of healthy eating and exercise to see very little, if any movement. This will cause the same mentality as we saw in the boxing example; it seems like a lot of effort for very little reward. It is easy to get fixated on details such as increments of measurement, even so far as worrying about as little as quarter of a pound. Instead, if you are going to gauge your success by weight or measurements, then it would be more advisable to only take these stats a minimum of once every four to six weeks. You are much more likely to see good results, which will help keep you motivated and help you recognize that the changes you are making are working.

**Emotional Motivation**

Our emotions play a huge part in what decisions we make on a day to day basis, which in turn impact on our health and wellbeing. Sometimes, we don't even realize that we are making bad decisions. They are simply disguised by the strength of our feelings at the time. It can be as simple as sitting in front of the television and finishing a whole bag of chips because you are bored. It could be that a bad day has you reaching for ice cream and cookies. It could even be that you feel stressed, so you don't eat anything all day, but then by the evening your body is crying out for energy. As a result, you choose all the wrong foods and go to bed on a very heavy stomach that is still working hard to digest everything you have binged on.

**Why does eating make us feel better?**

When we are experiencing a flood of emotions, eating may make us feel better, but it is only a short term response. It is due to the fact that eating stimulates a response from the gut, which in turn prompts our neurotransmitters to start making serotonin, a chemical that is vital for balancing our moods. The more serotonin the happier and more contented we feel.

Instead, it is much healthier to find natural ways to maintain or raise our serotonin levels. Ways we can do this include:

- Avoid caffeinated drinks, especially energy drinks. Caffeine suppresses serotonin which explains why it also inhibits our hunger.
- Eat healthy fats such as Omega 3 fatty acids, which can be found in oily fish, nuts, and seeds. They contain DHA which is an essential building block for brain function.
- Eat dark chocolate. As if we need an excuse! However, dark chocolate is very beneficial for your serotonin levels as it contains resveratrol, which boosts endorphins and serotonin levels.
- Eat wisely. Choose complex carbohydrates, such as whole grain bread and pasta. Whole grains take much longer to be absorbed by the body, meaning that the effects of eating – including serotonin production – last much longer.
- De-stress as much as possible! Prolonged periods of stress can seriously lower serotonin levels. Whether it is a hot bath or a yoga class, take time to chill out and relax.
- Exercise regularly. Exercise creates an increase in tryptophan, which is the precursor to serotonin and is present in the body even after the exercise is finished, suggesting a prolonged heightened mood.
- Get some sunshine. Natural sunlight is proven to help raise serotonin levels.

More and more people are identifying themselves as emotional eaters. That is they eat or don't eat depending on how they feel. Triggers are usually negative emotions and can include: anxiety, upset, stress, depression, and boredom. If this sounds like you, then you can use this as a motivational tool to help you kick the habit of emotional eating and get started on a healthier lifestyle.

The first step, once you have recognized the problem, is to accept it. Don't berate yourself about it; it is more common than you think. Blaming yourself will create more negative feelings, prompting you to seek comfort through food again. Instead, work on identifying your triggers for emotional eating. You can do this via a journal, writing down every time you feel the urge to snack and what you are feeling at the time. Make sure to note any specific cravings, too, for example; always wanting a candy bar mid-afternoon may be an indication of a slump in blood sugar levels. This can easily be remedied by swapping the candy bar for a juicy piece of fruit. Once you know the triggers for your emotional eating, you can work on having a plan in place to either avoid them or face them head on.

## Giving up smoking

If you smoke any sort of tobacco, giving up the habit is one of *the* most beneficial things you can do for your health. Many people believe that eating right and exercising is all they need to do to stay healthy, but smoking will undo all that effort and more.

We know you are probably sick of people telling you that you need to quit and it will be extremely hard, but there is plenty of help available to you if you reach out for it. We are not going to preach to you, but we will share some basic information that should help you make the decision that quitting smoking will be the best thing for your health.

The American Lung Association website states that 392,000 people in the US die every year from tobacco related diseases and another 50,000 die from conditions related to second-hand smoke exposure.

Here are some facts about what effect smoking is having on your body:

*Brain*

Smoking increases your risk of having a stroke by 50% or more. This is partly because you are more at risk of developing a brain aneurysm, which can cause brain damage and death.

If you were to stop smoking today, within two years, your risk is reduced to half that of a non-smoker and, within five years, you would have the same risk as a non-smoker.

*Circulation*

Toxins from cigarette smoke enter the blood stream and cause a number of problems including thickening your blood, which makes the chance of you developing a clot or DVT much higher. It will also narrow your arteries, meaning that the amount of blood circulating to your vital organs is slowed, and increase your heart rate and blood pressure, making your heart work much harder to keep your body functioning.

Again, these symptoms increase your risk of stroke or of having a heart attack.

## Heart

Smoking doubles the risk of you having a heart attack and smokers will have twice the risk of dying from heart disease. This is mostly due to the effect that smoking has on circulation as explained above.

If you were to stop smoking today, within a year, your risk of serious heart conditions is reduced by half.

## Lungs

84% of deaths from lung cancer and 83% of deaths from chronic obstructive lung disease are caused by smoking. Other chronic conditions include: emphysema, coughs, wheezing, and asthma.

Within days of stopping smoking, you will begin to see a positive effect on this area of your health.

## Mouth/Throat

More than 93% of throat cancers are caused by smoking and cancers can be found in the lips, tongue, voice box, throat, and oesophagus.

Stopping smoking will greatly reduce the chance of developing this type of cancer and, after twenty years, your risks will reduce to that of a non-smoker.

## Stomach

Those who smoke are increasing the likelihood of developing ulcers and acid reflux due to a weakening of the muscle at the base of the oesophagus. Also, you are more at risk of developing kidney cancer and are twice as likely to develop it if you smoke twenty or more cigarettes a day.

As you can see, there is huge medical evidence to support the damage that smoking can do to not only your health, but also to that of the people who are regularly around you when you smoke.

There are numerous methods available to help you quit, including nicotine patches, lozenges, inhalers, and sprays; as well as stronger medication. You may also like to consider some of the alternative techniques including: hypnotherapy and acupuncture.

For advice on how to get started, contact your doctor or pharmacist. They may also be able to point you in the direction of a local support group where you can speak to others who are also hoping to quit. For more information you can check out: http://smokefree.gov/

Good luck, you can do it!

**Getting Started**

*"Something is better than nothing".*

While this saying may not sound like the most motivational, ass-kicking start to your new healthy lifestyle, the first thing to remember is that you need to start off with small, sustainable changes. If you attempt to change everything right away and at one time, you are much more likely to fail and you cannot expect to be able to change bad habits overnight. This piece of advice is especially true if you are embarking on exercise after leading a relatively sedentary lifestyle, as overdoing it can cause more harm than good. There will be a lot more information on getting moving and getting active in Chapter 9.

Examples of some small, positive changes that you could make at the start of your journey include:

- Making sure you eat breakfast every day
- Getting off the bus one stop earlier and walking
- Eating five portions of fruits and vegetables a day
- Taking the stairs at work
- Drinking at least eight glasses / two liters of water per day
- Walk to the local grocery store instead of driving
- Swap your nightly glass of white wine for red
- Take the batteries out of the remote and get up to change the channel

These illustrate some very simple, yet effective ways you can start to develop healthy habits. Remember, it can take up to a month to make a change to a habit, so if you start today, in thirty days time these small changes will be second nature.

More information on healthy food and exercise will be covered in later chapters of the book.

## Reward Yourself!

There is no sense putting in all this effort if you don't occasionally reward yourself, but it's *how* you reward yourself that is important. Whereas before you may have treated yourself to a takeaway, a bar of chocolate, or a bottle of wine, you can find new, original, and healthy ways to treat yourself instead, all it takes is a little imagination! You can even set weekly or monthly goals as added motivation. For example; "If I go to the gym at least six times this month, I will reward myself with a day at the spa." Alternatively, treat yourself to some new trainers, a smoothie-maker, a trial at a new gym, or some new bedding. Anything that is beneficial to your new lifestyle makes an ideal reward.

## Buddy Up!

Support can be invaluable when you are looking to change your lifestyle and it makes it so much more fun when you have a buddy that you can talk to, swap ideas with, and lean on the days where you are finding it tough. Speak to your doctor or have a look online and see if there are any local support groups near you. Joining fitness classes can also be a great way to make new friends who will help you on your journey.

## Nobody is Perfect!

This is vitally important to remember. You are only human and there will be days where you may fall off the wagon and give in to temptation. What matters is that you don't use that as an excuse to fall back into your old habits, but instead you draw a line under it and get back on plan. One bad meal, one bad day, or even a weekend doesn't have to mean the end of the healthy new you. Just look back on how far you have already come to motivate you.

## Get some sleep!

Sleep is a vital part of having a healthy body and mind as it affects many of our day to day functions. Sleep deprivation has known links to mood swings, depression, and difficulty in controlling emotions. Being tired, and therefore irritable, is a key trigger for emotional eating, particularly if we are craving carbohydrate-heavy foods to provide us with energy.

Sleep is the time in which our bodies heal and repair themselves. This is why many seriously injured or sick people are put into medically-induced comas, as it allows their bodies to be much more efficient in the healing process. Lack of sleep can affect our immune systems, blood sugar levels, and digestive process among other things.

While the optimum amount of sleep for a person can vary, a rough estimate is between seven and nine hours per night. Make sure you establish a calming bedtime routine and skip any caffeinated drinks after 6:00 p.m. to help you get a restful night of good quality sleep.

**Negativity**

*"Do it because they said you couldn't".*

Anyone that cares about you and your wellbeing should be happy to support you in your journey to create a better, healthier lifestyle. However, sadly there are still plenty of people that love to try and spread negativity. This is often a result of jealousy or because they may have failed where you are succeeding. If you have had a particularly unhealthy lifestyle before now, they may ridicule your ability to change at all. There are countless other reasons why someone may be negative about the steps that you are taking. It can be very disheartening and even hurtful when it happens, but there is something you can do that will make you feel better, use it to motivate you.

Do you remember as a child when your parents would tell you that you couldn't have something and it just made you want it all the more? Or when someone told you that you couldn't climb that tree because you were too small, but you did it anyway? *That* is the kind of motivation that you need to take from any negativity you are shown for your decisions to become a healthy human being. Just make sure that you remember that you are doing it for you and your family, no-one else.

*"It doesn't really matter who I used to be. All that matters is who I have become".*

We hope that you have found this chapter motivational and informative as you begin to make the changes that you need in order to embrace a new, healthier and more natural lifestyle. During this chapter, we have looked at what motivates you to change; whether it is physical, emotional or otherwise, and we have given you some suggestions as to what you can do to combat any challenges that threaten this motivation. We have touched on the importance of giving up smoking and rounded off with a few suggestions and hints to help you on your way.

In the next chapter, it is going to be all about food. We are going to explain why meal planning is a key step of healthy eating and why it is important to always be prepared. We are going to help you understand how to make healthy food choices and give you some example meal plans and shopping lists. Most importantly we are going to demonstrate that eating healthy doesn't mean going hungry!

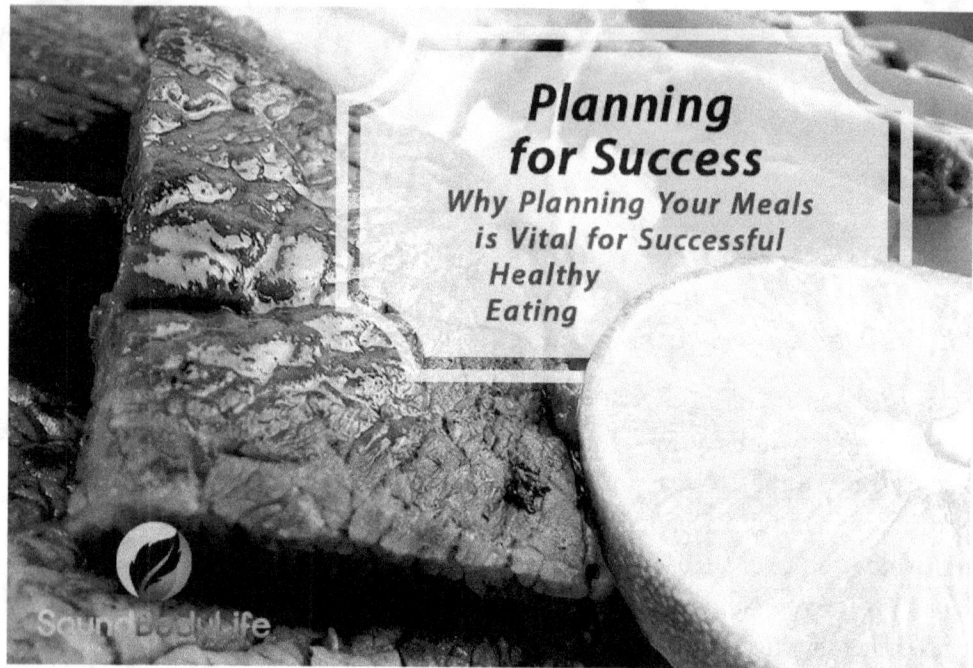

# Chapter 7

*Planning
for Success*
*Why Planning Your Meals
is Vital for Successful
Healthy
Eating*

Food plays a critical part of a healthy lifestyle, but increasingly hectic schedules, tiredness, and laziness all contribute to us making the wrong food choices. It can feel so tempting to order a pizza after a long day at work or grab a packet of crisps out of the cupboard when we are bored. However, these bad food choices are contributing to obesity, chronic health conditions, and even premature death. That is why this chapter is going to focus on food and the importance of not only planning our meals, but preparing for the unexpected. We are going to help you understand how you can easily make healthy food choices and show you some tips for not succumbing to temptation. We are also going to give you some example meal plans to get you started.

## Meal Planning

Meal planning is a strange concept to a lot of people who consider it 'nerdish' and 'dull', but in actual fact it can save you a lot of time, energy, and money. It will also ultimately improve your eating habits and reduce the likelihood of you making unhealthy meal choices.

So, what is meal planning? Well, it is exactly what it suggests, planning your meals in advance, including your snacks. How far in advance you want to plan them is entirely up to you. Meal planning is a very personal thing and what works for you and your family may not work at all for somebody else. Some people plan for up to a month at a time, doing one large shopping trip and freezing as much as possible. Other people stock up on the pantry basics and then shop for fresh meat on a daily basis, although many say that they find that increased trips to the store means increased spending on items that they don't really need. If you opt for frequent trips for shopping, then you need to try and stick completely to the list that you take with you. However, what is most important about meal planning is that you find a method that works for you.

# What are the benefits of meal planning?

- You will make better food choices

Meal planning will help you make better food choices and stick to them. This is because you will be limiting the number of decisions that you need to make each day and, as such, you will be less likely to be influenced by externals factors that might make you opt for unhealthy convenience food. For example; imagine that you know that you always go to the movies straight from work on a Thursday and you don't normally get home until 8pm. By the time you get home, you are usually tired from the day and the last thing that you feel like doing is preparing a meal. Instead, it becomes easier to just stop and pick up a takeaway on the way home. Not only does this become a costly habit, but invariably it becomes an unhealthy one, too, as most restaurants and take-outs fail to provide healthy and nutritious food. Similarly, pre-packaged and microwaveable meals can be just as bad, being so processed that any nutritional value is lost.

Now, if you know that you are usually late home on a Thursday, you can prepare for this and that is the key to meal planning – preparation. Knowing this fact about a specific night of the week, you can take steps such as pre-preparing a meal that you can either eat cold from the refrigerator or a home-made dinner that just needs heating. This takes the decision making process out of your hands and you know that you can eat a healthy, nutritious meal with minimum effort that evening.

- You will shop more efficiently

Meal planning removes some of the spontaneity that often creeps into grocery shopping. It is so easy to be tempted by special offers and discounts, meaning that we often buy far more than we need. You will also find that the majority of discounts are usually found on unhealthy items, as they are products that are cheap for stores to buy. Remember, quality food negates a quality price tag!

Planning your meals in advance will mean that it is absolutely necessary to create a list before you go. You will know exactly what meals you will need and can write down the components and ingredients that you will have to shop for in accordance with this. This will also help to eliminate food waste as you can be sure that you will use everything that you have purchased, rather than buying groceries because you think you will eat them at some point, but instead they are left languishing in the freezer or at the back of the pantry.

- You will save money

There is something gut-wrenching about throwing away spoiled food, especially when so many people in the world are hungry. We have said that meal planning will reduce or eliminate food waste and this, in turn, will save you money. It will also reduce the amount of money that you spend on takeaways which are generally expensive, charging people for the convenience as well as the food that they consume.

Having a regular meal plan will also allow you to shop around for the best value ingredients for your dishes, meaning that you can make your money stretch even further. It will also allow you to budget more effectively, as you will know exactly what you will need to buy to cover all of the meals for a specific time period.

- Bulk-cooking & freezing

Some meals, such as cottage pie or bolognaise can be made in bulk and frozen to be used as meals at a later date. This is especially useful if you know you are unlikely to want to cook one evening, like in our previous example. Frozen home-made meals can be cooked easily and quickly, making eating a nutritious meal simple and not at all time consuming. Many people keep spare batches of healthy home-made dinners in their freezer, well labelled with the date that they are frozen, to act as fall-backs if plans change unexpectedly. That way they know that they will always have a good meal choice available.

- Varied nutrition

Planning your meals also allows you to choose food that will provide a wide range of nutritional content. This means you and your family can be sure you receive all the vitamins, minerals, and other goodness that you need to maintain a healthy body and mind.

- Development of healthy habits

Breaking bad habits and making healthy ones can be very hard, especially if you are surrounded by temptation when you make decisions about what and when to eat. Meal planning can remove a lot of the decision making process; for example, you may opt to have home-made tacos on a Friday night. Before long this will replace a previously unhealthy habit, such as ordering pizza on a Friday night. Development of healthy habits is vital to maintaining a successfully healthy lifestyle. Even small changes, such as always drinking a pint of water before dinner or not skipping breakfast, can make a big difference.

Guidelines for good eating habits:

1. Maintain a regular eating routine
2. Fill up of healthy, natural foods
3. Eat slowly and once you are full, stop!
4. Snack on fruit, vegetables, and nuts/seeds
5. Choose whole grains & high fibre foods
6. Drink at least 8 glasses of water every day

## Getting started with meal planning

So, how do you get started? It's easy; grab a pen and paper to write down what your favorite meals are. At this point, if you are also going to be preparing food for a partner or other family members, it is important to take their opinions into account, too. That way it will make it much easier to please everyone and prevent you from having to make more than one meal per evening. Even if some of the meals appear quite unhealthy or some of them are takeaways foods, include them in the list.

Now work through the list, writing down the ingredients that you will need to make each dish. For takeaway foods, find recipes online to make the same thing at home. For example; if you particularly like beef in oyster sauce from the Chinese takeaway, have a look online for simple recipes that you can replicate at home using lower calorie and healthier ingredients. It will also be possible for you to swap out many of the ingredients for normal home-cooked meals to make them lower calorie and more nutritious. Here are some examples for you, but you could also visit the grocery store and look online for more ideas.

- When making cream-based sauces, swap full fat for reduced fat cream.
- When using strongly-flavored cheese in dishes, you can normally reduce the amount used without compromising on flavor. Alternatively opt for low-fat cheese.
- Cooking fat can add an awful lot of calories to our meals which is a shame as they are only for purpose rather than taste. Instead of using solid fat or vegetable oils, swap for olive oil or low fat cooking sprays which are healthier.
- Red meat can contain a lot of fat, but it is possible to purchase low-fat varieties or leaner cuts. Once you have browned the meat, drain it to remove any excess fat before continuing cooking.
- Swap chicken for turkey sometimes. Turkey is much lower in fat than chicken.
- Look for low-fat versions of butter, mayonnaise, and other dressings. They are often lower in calories as well as saturated and Trans fats, making them an overall healthier choice.
- Vegetables that are covered in cream, butter, or cheese sauces add heaps of extra calories to a meal. Instead, pick up fresh or frozen vegetables such as green beans, asparagus, and broccoli that you can steam in the microwave, giving you all the nutrition and taste without putting extra calories on to your plate.
- Adding dry beans to some entrees and soups can be a great way to extend the recipe and add nutritional value. This is especially easy to do in chili and vegetable soups as canned kidney, pinto, or white beans make a great accompaniment to the dish. Similarly, black beans can be added to Mexican-style meals such as enchiladas and burritos.

## Meals on the Run

Life is hectic and there is always going to be times where we will need to grab something to eat whilst rushing around. Whether it is breakfast, lunch, or snacks and whether you are in the car, at your desk, or somewhere else, food on the go doesn't have to be unhealthy. Filling and nutritious examples include:

- High-protein snacks such as low-fat turkey slices or a variety of nuts and seeds.
- Whole-grain crackers and bread.
- Low-fat or fat-free dairy products like natural yoghurt, low-fat cheese and skimmed milk.
- Fresh vegetables. Carrot batons, pepper sticks, celery and cucumber all make filling and nutritious snacks and go great with a low-fat dip.
- Fruit. Most fruit is ready to eat and bananas, apples, pears, peaches, and grapes are all easy to transport and mess-free to eat. You can also opt for dried fruit like raisins.

When you make your grocery list each week, make sure you do a thorough stock check to see what healthy snacks you need. Keep a stock of them in your car, desk, or cupboards to help you resist the urge to reach for the chips or chocolate. You will find it much easier to stick to your new healthier diet when you have a variety of delicious and nutritious foods on hand.

## Helpful planning hints

Everyone will need to plan their meals differently based upon a variety of factors. These include how many people we are cooking for, where we shop, and, of course, what our schedules are. Bear in mind that many of these factors are also variable. Perhaps your partner works away part of the week so you only have to cook for yourself some days or perhaps you usually have friends for dinner on a Friday evening. You may find that one week you require more quick and easy evening meals due to a change in your schedule. This is why it is important to review your meal plan on a weekly basis to ensure that all circumstances are covered with your new healthy food choices.

## Your schedule

Paying attention to your schedule is absolutely critical for effective meal planning. You need to know how much time you have to both prepare and eat your meals each day and, of course, this may vary considerably. When you do your planning, take both of these into account. It can be very handy to vary your meals throughout the week, alternating between those that require more preparation and those that are quick and easy or involve leftovers, and structuring your plan to fit these in on the appropriate days in your schedule. Using a slow cooker is also a viable option on the days where preparation and cooking time is limited.

It can also be helpful to have a 'back-up' meal stored in the freezer in case you have a day where things don't go quite to plan. Then you don't need to forfeit your good lifestyle and be tempted to make a phone call to the takeaway!

## Be careful with bargain hunting

Let's face it, most of us have a budget when it comes to shopping, but when we are faced with a bargain, we can be tempted to make a purchase without really knowing when or how we are going to use it. Impulse food purchases are major contributors to food (and money!) going to waste. However, you can still grab a bargain if you factor coupons, deals, and sales into the planning stage of your shopping. If you know you have specific coupons to use that week or your grocery store has sales on particular foods, just work out what meals you can incorporate those products into. A deal for $2 off chicken breasts? Simply check your schedule and see when you have enough time to make a meal using chicken breasts; for example, you may be able to cook chicken fajitas on Thursday evening. Planning what dish you are going to make first means that you can take up the offers that are worthwhile, saving you money and reducing the risk of food waste. Then simply add the other ingredients that you will need to your shopping list.

Don't forget though, a bargain is not a bargain if it is for an unhealthy product. Most coupons tend to be for highly processed foods. If it is for a product that isn't nutritious, then you are better off putting the coupon straight in the bin, that way you won't be tempted to use it for the sake of a good deal!

*Source seasonal produce*

Fruits and vegetables that are in season are usually cheaper and much more readily available. Filling up on these items is also a great way to boost nutritional value in your diet, so it is well worth choosing fruits and vegetables that are in season and planning your meals in accordance.

*Organize your recipes*

Recipe books are fantastic, but the format in which ingredients and methods are laid out can sometimes be confusing and tricky to follow. When it comes to planning your meals, you may find it beneficial to copy our recipes that you plan to use. By doing so, you can use the same template for all recipes, making it simpler for you to see exactly what you need and what process to follow. This will make writing your shopping lists much easier as you refer to it. Write each recipe onto a separate sheet of paper and pop them in a binder, organizing them by parameters to suit your requirements.

*Get a chalkboard or whiteboard*

Having a chalkboard or whiteboard in your kitchen can be an invaluable part of meal planning, particularly as it is so easy to lose pieces of paper between writing down and needing them. Each time you run out of something, write it down. This will prevent you from starting a recipe that you cannot finish because you have run out of a specific ingredient and remind you what needs to be added to the grocery list. If you finish a jar or packet of something, then be sure to write it on the list before you throw it in the garbage, otherwise distractions mean that you will likely forget. You can also use this technique to replace other household goods such as toilet paper and cleaning products.

*Create a master grocery list*

Unlocking the secrets to successful meal planning requires a key and that key is organization. There are certain items such as bread, milk, and eggs that you will likely need to buy every time you do your grocery shop. It is helpful to have a generic list already in place that includes these staple items. Not only will it save time, but it will stop you overlooking the obvious things when it comes to making your list. You can then add in items from your white/chalkboard that need replacing, followed by the specific ingredients that you need to make the dishes on your meal plan.

## Tips from some Food Experts

**1. Make the commitment.** The first step to healthier eating is commitment to your plan, says Susan Nicholson, author of the syndicated newspaper column *7 Day Menu Planner*. Make the decision and then stick with it, and get your family to support you by getting them involved in the planning process.

**2. Pick a plan to suit your lifestyle.** "I love the 'cook once, eat twice' strategy," says Ellie Krieger, RD, host of *Healthy Appetite* on the Food Network and author of *The Food You Crave*.

"I plan my weekly meals by first deciding what three major proteins I'm going to eat, and then I make them do double duty. If I buy a rotisserie chicken, I prepare a salad one night and chicken tacos the next. If I'm making roasted pork loin with veggies on Monday, I may use the leftover for pulled-pork sandwiches Wednesday night."

Susan Nicholson opts for planning for four weeks of menus on a calendar or grid. For each day, she lists an entrée, sides, and dessert, and highlights any days that she routinely eats away from home. "Most of us have at least 10 favorite meals. If you're a beginner, it's simple to fill in those 10 then repeat them until the grid is full." When you're ready, start adding new recipes or tweak your menu to keep things fresh and interesting.

**3. Make a shopping list.** Keep a generic list that includes things you buy frequently (such as milk, eggs, chicken breasts), and then include the additional things to make the meals on your plan so you don't have to start from scratch each week, Susan Nicholson says. She puts a shopping-list template on her computer and arranges ingredients in sections to correspond with the layout of her regular supermarket to make shopping easier and more methodical.

**4. Shop strategically.** "Shop on a day that works best for you," says Toni Lydecker, author of *Serves One: Simple Meals to Savor When You're on Your Own*. If you seem to always shop at a time when the shelves are depleted, consider asking your store when it receives fresh shipments from vendors. Be flexible with your list, too. If you're planning to cook green beans one night, but the asparagus looks fresher, choose that instead.

**5. Cook perishable produce first.** "Cook with perishables like fresh fish or salad greens early in the week," Toni Lydecker also advises. "Then later you can rely on staples: a simple omelet or pasta dish."

Ellie Krieger prefers to balance her grocery purchases with a variety of fresh and frozen produce. "It's easy to overdo it on the fresh produce and end up throwing out extras," she says. She opts for frozen vegetables like peas, spinach, and corn to use on days when her supplies of fresh produce have run low.

**6. Review your meals to see what works.** "Every time you finish a meal, critique it," Susan Nicholson recommends. "When a meal works, give it a gold star." Keep a track of your gold-star meals so menu planning takes less time. In just a few weeks, you'll have a complete collection of time-tested and family-approved meals.

## Sample Meal Plans

If the idea of planning your meals is still a little daunting, we have sourced and adapted some sample meal plans that you can use to give you examples of what you should be looking to create in order to get started.

| Week One | Menu | Ingredients | Cupboard Staples |
|---|---|---|---|
| SUNDAY | Grilled chicken tenderloin<br><br>Grilled asparagus<br><br>Corn and roasted red peppers<br><br>Baked potato | Approx 2.5lbs of chicken tenderloin (enough for leftovers for Tuesday)<br><br>Asparagus<br><br>Baking Potatoes<br><br>Frozen corn<br><br>2 red peppers | Olive oil |
| MONDAY | Black beans and rice<br><br>Coleslaw | 2 cans black beans<br><br>1 can of tomatoes<br><br>Frozen corn<br><br>1 large head of green | Brown rice<br><br>Hot sauce<br><br>Cumin |

| | | cabbage | Cider vinegar |
|---|---|---|---|
| | | 1 mid-size jalapeno pepper | Olive oil |
| | | | Garlic powder |
| | | Green onions | Chopped garlic |
| | | | Oregano |
| | | | Cilantro |
| | | | Onion |
| TUESDAY | Garden Salad | Lettuce | Whole wheat pasta shells |
| | Wholegrain Parmesan toast | Cherry tomatoes | 100% wholegrain bread |
| | Melon | Cucumber | |
| | | Carrots | Parmesan cheese |
| | | Leftover turkey (from Sunday) | |
| | | Cantaloupe Melon | |
| WEDNESDAY | Baked fish with pineapple salsa | Fish | Skimmed milk |
| | Broccoli bake | 2 cups of pineapple chunks | Onion |
| | Steamed carrots | 1 red pepper | Cilantro |
| | | 1-2 jalapeño peppers | Breadcrumbs |
| | | 3 cups of frozen chopped broccoli | Whole wheat |
| | | Carrots | Whole wheat pasta spirals |
| | | 1 10oz can of low fat cream of broccoli soup | |
| THURSDAY | Cabbage roll | 1lb lean ground beef | Brown rice |
| | Apple and beet salad | 1 14oz can of crushed tomatoes | |
| | | Cabbage (leftover from Monday) | |

| | | 1 can of beets | |
| | | Radishes | |
| | | Scallions | |
| | | 4 Granny Smith apples | |
| | | Apple juice | |
| FRIDAY | Vegetarian chili with spinach <br><br> Cornbread | Cornbread mix <br><br> 1 can of chili-style beans <br><br> 1 can of pinto beans <br><br> 1 can of unsalted stewed tomatoes <br><br> 4oz of frozen spinach | Brown rice |
| SATURDAY | Spaghetti with quick tomato sauce <br><br> Mixed salad <br><br> Wholegrain bread with roasted garlic | 2 cans of crushed tomatoes <br><br> Parmesan cheese <br><br> Cherry tomatoes <br><br> Lettuce <br><br> Shredded carrots <br><br> Cucumber <br><br> Radishes | Spaghetti <br><br> Garlic <br><br> Parmesan cheese <br><br> Garlic <br><br> Onion <br><br> Wholegrain bread |

## Low-Calorie Sample Day Menus

| 1200 Calories | | |
| --- | --- | --- |
| **Breakfast** | **Lunch** | **Dinner** |
| 0.5 Grapefruit <br> 1 slice Whole Wheat Bread <br> 1 cup (8oz) Milk (skim, nonfat) | 2 slices Rye Bread <br> 2oz Turkey Breast <br> 2 stalks of Celery <br> 1 Carrot <br> 1 tbsp Ranch (fat free) <br> 1 Peach <br> 1 cup Milk (skim, nonfat) | Bouillon <br> 1 Parsley Potato (2-in diameter) <br> 3 oz Roast Veal, lean <br> 0.5 cup Peas & Carrots <br> 1 Green Salad <br> 2 tsp Salad dressing <br> 0.5 cup Applesauce (unsweetened) |

## 1500 Calories

| Breakfast | Lunch | Dinner |
|---|---|---|
| 12 oz. Coffee (w/ caffeine)<br>1 cup Milk (skim)<br>1 package Instant Oatmeal<br>1 Orange | 2 slices Whole Wheat Bread<br>2 oz. Turkey Breast (white, low sodium)<br>0.5 cup Alfalfa Sprouts<br>0.2 cup Tomato<br>1 cubic inch Cheddar Cheese<br>0.2 cup Lettuce | 5 oz. Tilapia<br>0.25 cup Fresh Cilantro<br>1 cup Steamed Brown Rice<br>0.5 cup Mixed Steamed Broccoli<br>& Yellow Squash<br>1 small Salad<br>2 tbsp Fat Free Dressing |

## 1800 Calories

| Breakfast | Lunch | Dinner |
|---|---|---|
| 1 cup Milk (skim)<br>1 c Strawberries (fresh)<br>1 Bagel (whole wheat or bran)<br>2 tbsp Cream Cheese (fat free)<br>0.1 c raisins (seedless) | Lunch 1 cup Cranberry Juice (light)<br>1 Whole Wheat Pita<br>3 oz. Light Tuna (in water)<br>1 tbsp Mayo (light)<br>0.25 cup sliced Tomato<br>0.2 cup Spinach Leaves (raw)<br>1 medium Orange | 4 oz. Chicken Breast (white meat)<br>1 tbsp Lemon Juice (fresh)<br>1 tbsp Ground Pepper (fresh)<br>1 small Sweet Potato (baked)<br>1 small Salad<br>0.2 cup cucumber<br>0.2 cup diced tomato<br>0.2 cup diced sweet peppers<br>1 tbsp lemon juice<br>1 tsp parsley (dried)<br>1 small Whole Wheat Roll |

## 2200 Calories

| Breakfast | Lunch | Dinner |
|---|---|---|
| 3 Egg White Omelette<br>2 tbsp chopped green peppers<br>1 tbsp chopped onion<br>2 tbsp chopped tomato<br>2 tsp Canola Oil (if needed)<br>1 cup Milk (skim, nonfat)<br>1 slice Whole Wheat Toast<br>1 tbsp Almond Butter (w/o salt)<br>0.5 cup cubed Cantaloupe/Melon | 2 cup Spinach (raw)<br>2 oz. Skinless Chicken Breast (not fried; roasted, baked, etc.)<br>2 tbsp Black Bean & Corn Salsa (instead of salad dressing)<br>2 tbsp shredded Mexican Blend Cheese (0.25c)<br>1 sesame Bread stick<br>1 cup nonfat skim milk<br>1 orange | 4 oz. broiled salmon (wild)<br>1 cup couscous<br>0.75 cup broccoli<br>0.75 cup carrots<br>Tomato & Mozzarella<br>1 cup tomato slices 0.5 cup low sodium mozzarella |

We hope that this chapter has demonstrated how important planning your meals is to your new healthy lifestyle. Without a plan in place, it is so easy to give in to the temptation of convenience food, which is almost always unhealthy and lacking in any real nutrition or goodness. We have explained how to use your weekly schedule in order to make a truly workable plan and why you should consider keeping fall-back meals just in case things somehow go wrong. We have also shared some tips for preparing your grocery list and how to get the most out of supermarket deals.

In the next chapter, we are going to accompany you to our virtual grocery store where we help you shop for your groceries. We are going to look at what foods you should be filling on and what foods you should be avoiding. We are also going to explore the minefield that is grocery labeling, helping you to decipher the jargon which will allow you to make informed choices. Finally, we are going to share with you our very best tips and tricks to help you stick firmly to plan and avoid the temptations that will be lurking in every aisle. Read on to learn how to make every trip to the grocery store a healthy and nutritious one.

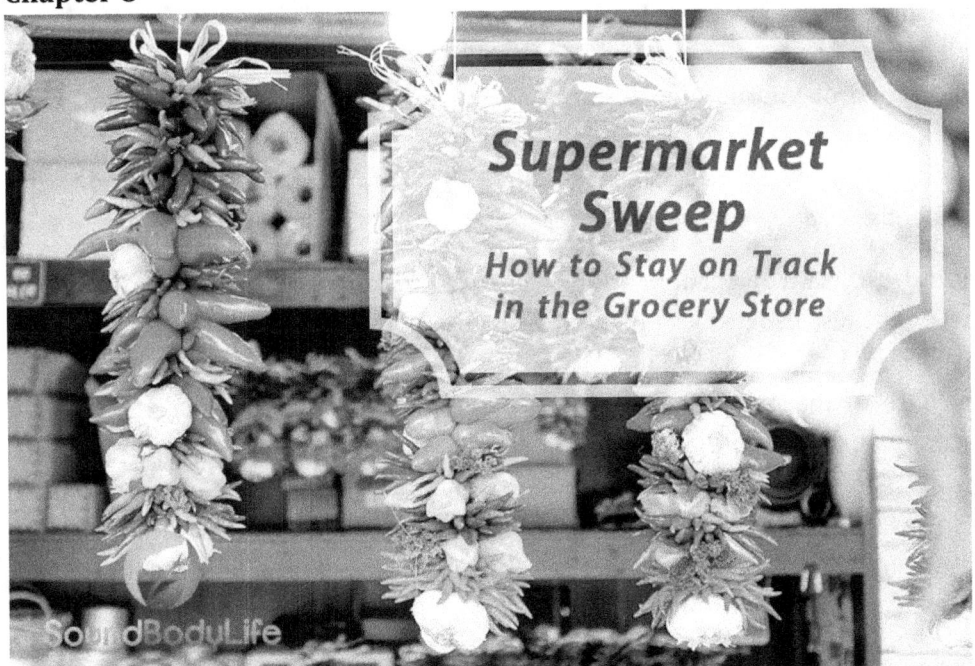

# Chapter 8

## Supermarket Sweep
### How to Stay on Track in the Grocery Store

Going to the supermarket can be overwhelming, distracting, and very tempting, especially if you o shopping when you are already feeling hungry. One of the key reasons for impulse purchases when doing the grocery shopping is a rumbling stomach. When we are feeling hungry, we are more likely to pick up food that would be a quick, energy-providing, and filling fix. As we have learned, that usually comes in the form of simple carbohydrates which we know are not at all good for us. They will give us a short burst of energy and fill us up temporarily, but before long the hunger pangs will kick in again. So, one of the most important pieces of advice that we could give you regarding your trips to the store is to make sure that you never, ever go when you are feeling hungry!

During this chapter, we are going to visit our virtual grocery store where we will help you navigate the aisles to select good, nutritious food and avoid the bad. We are also going to look at how to unravel the jargon found on labels so we can decipher which foods truly are good for you and which are unhealthy products in disguise. We are going to give you our top tricks and ideas for tackling the supermarket to ensure that you stick to your plan.

## Planning ahead

During Chapter 7, we covered the importance of meal planning and how it is a vital part of changing to a healthier lifestyle. Not only will it reduce the likelihood of you needing to buy convenience food, it will also give you the opportunity to ensure that you are eating all of the foods that you need to give you good health, which includes getting the optimum amount of vitamins and minerals.

Elizabeth Ward, the author of *The Pocket Idiot's Guide to Food Pyramids*, recommends using the guidelines featured on the government's nutrition website www.mypyramid.gov, to ensure that you are planning a harmonious balance of the nutrients that we need. Ward states that in order to fulfil the requirements of the pyramid, we should be filling our baskets primarily with fruits, vegetables, dairy, whole grains, poultry, lean meats, fish, nuts, and beans. However, we should try and incorporate variety too; for example, rather than always choosing plain potatoes, try and swap for sweet potatoes, which are a greater source of beta-carotene.

Once you have your plans made and your shopping list written it is time to head for the supermarket.

## Aisle by Aisle checklist

### Fresh produce

In the majority of supermarkets, the very first area you will encounter will be the fresh produce. It is designed to entice customers with its bright colours and fresh aroma. You may have heard people say that colourful foods are healthier and this is absolutely the case. There is something much more inviting about a plate of vibrant food than a plate of bland browns and yellows. The colours actually reflect the different minerals, vitamins, and phytonutrients that are present in each fruit or vegetable.

Needless to say that this stuff should be the staple of your diet. Whatever you decide to put with them and however you decide to cook, dress, or serve them, fresh fruit and vegetables should make up a large proportion of your shopping cart.

## Meat, fish and poultry

Two servings of fish per week is the amount that is recommended by The American Heart Association. Salmon is one of the most popular choices because it is affordable, widely available, and a fantastic source of Omega-3 fatty acids, which are essential for good health. Meat is packed with protein, which provides us with longer and more sustainable energy levels. However, try and ensure that you pick lean cuts of meat, such as tenderloin, and cut away any thick layers of fat. If you choose to eat poultry, you should remember to remove all of the skin before consumption, as it is extremely fatty.

## Breads, pasta and cereal

The important thing to remember with these food groups is to always choose the least processed option and always pick whole grains. Whole grains, as we know, offer complex carbohydrates, which make us feel fuller for longer. They are considerably better for our health, containing far less sugar and much more fibre. When choosing whole-grain cereals, try and pick one that has a minimum of four grams of fibre and the lowest amount of sugar possible.

1 level teaspoon of sugar = four grams of sugar

If you have fussy children (or adults!) in your family that object to the flavour of whole grains, you could start by introducing mixed blends until they start to adapt before eventually making the transition to a 100% whole grain lifestyle.

You should also be aware of very cleverly disguised cereal bars. Many which are marketed as being a healthy choice are actually very high in sugar, additives, and other unhealthy elements. This is also seen in many 'flavoured porridges' as the addition of sweeteners, such as maple syrup, also mean the addition of sugar.

## Dairy

Vitamin D and calcium are two vital nutrients provided by dairy products and they are vital for good health and, in particular, strong bones. This is one reason why growing children are encouraged to drink milk. Three servings of dairy per day is recommended, but there are plenty of low or non-fat choices available to help you keep calories and fat intake low. Examples include: yoghurts, yoghurt drinks and pre-portioned size cheeses. If you prefer the taste of full-fat dairy, then it is not off-limits. Just remember to keep your portion sizes relatively small.

### Dried or canned produce

Most pantries or cupboards are stocked with some staple dried or canned produce as they tend to have a long shelf life. Tins of vegetables and beans are great to bulk out meals such as soups, salads, and rice or pasta dishes. Tinned fruits can make a healthy dessert or even as a stand-alone snack. Check the labels and try to choose fruit that is in its own juice rather than syrup to cut out unnecessary sugar and opt for vegetables without any added salt. Low-fat soups, olive and canola oil, nut butters, tuna in water rather than brine, and assorted vinegars should be staple products for your cooking.

### Frozen food

During the winter months, it can be problematic trying to get hold of fresh produce. Whilst a lot of frozen foods are unhealthy mass-produced rubbish, it is possible to source some quality natural fruits and vegetables to fill your cupboards and refrigerator during the 'off' season, meaning that you can have a plentiful supply of the good stuff all year round. Other recommended frozen foods include plain low-fat cheese pizzas which you can load with vegetables, portion-controlled bagels, and whole grain waffles.

### Food in disguise

Food is generally divided into two categories: primarily healthy or primarily unhealthy. Sometimes we pick things that we believe are good for us, but in actual fact whilst they may not be unhealthy, there are far better nutrient-packed alternatives instead. However, thanks to some clever and pretty packaging, deceptive labelling, and some hidden ingredients, it can be very tricky to decipher which product is the better option. Here are ten food items that are often mistakenly considered to be the healthiest choice.

## 1. Iceberg lettuce

The crunch of iceberg lettuce is hugely appealing to consumers who find it tasty and refreshing. The reality is that it has far less nutritional value than the darker, leafy salads. The rule of thumb is that the darker the leaves are, the more nutrition it can provide.

## 2. Yoghurt covered nuts and pretzels

These are particularly popular with the under 16s age demographic, but the yoghurt that makes up these products is packed with unhealthy sugars and fat. When it is possible, always decide to purchase plain nuts and pretzels, with no added salts or sugars.

## 3. Fat-free dressings

Dressings that advertise themselves as 'fat free' often compensate for the lack of fat with other elements such as added sugar. For example, if you were to look at the label for fat-free yoghurt, you will likely see that it may contain only traces amounts of fat, but instead has more than twenty grams of sugar. We have already looked at the negative effects of sugar on the body and so such yoghurt is a primarily unhealthy food disguised as a healthy one.

You should not be aiming to cut all fat from your diet as this is too extreme and poses its own health problems. Some fat is necessary to help the body effectively absorb vital antioxidants and other vitamins.

## 4. Fruit-bottomed yoghurt

Whilst we are on the subject of yoghurt, many people believe that by selecting the varieties with fruit on the bottom, they are making a healthier choice. Unfortunately, these yoghurts are absolutely crammed full of sugars, flavourings, syrup, and a whole host of artificial ingredients.

### 5. Vanilla soy milk

Soy is another product that is often portrayed as the choice of healthy, nutritionally aware individuals. However, it too is actually loaded with additional sugar. Instead opt for regular unsweetened milk.

### 6. Pre-prepared packaged fruit

When faced with needing a snack on the run, you may think that grabbing a pot of pre-prepared fruit is making the right decision. Whilst it is undoubtedly healthier and more nutritious than chocolate or a bag of chips, pre-cut fruit usually suffers from some nutrient loss due to oxygen exposure when it was cut. It is also considerably more expensive thanks to costs incurred from packaging and preparing. To save yourself some money and give your body a real boost of vitamins and minerals, pick up a banana or an apple instead.

### 7. Bottled smoothies

Smoothies are a very popular way of getting your five (or more!) a day and has become a fashionable drink in recent years. Large supermarkets and other manufacturers have recognised this and brought out their own versions of smoothies. They tempt us with bright labels, promises of good nutrition, and convenience. However, yet again, many are artificially sweetened or full of nutritionally poor juices from pears and apples. It is much more cost effective and nutritionally beneficial to make your own.

### 8. Salted nuts and seeds

Some nuts, and particularly peanuts, have substantial amounts of fat. They are also high in salt which can increase your blood pressure and lead to heart disease.

## 9. Sweetened dried fruits

Again, we often think dried fruits are a good choice of snack. However, check the label carefully as many varieties have been sweetened before being packaged.

## 10. Vegetable oils

These heavily refined oils are usually made from soybean, cotton seed, or corn and are rich in omega-6 fatty acids which are responsible for inflammatory diseases. Olive oil or cooking sprays are a much healthier alternative.

**Some helpful shopping hints from Nestle**

Nestle have offered these top tips for helping to be supermarket smart.

- Avoid eating foods that contain more than five different ingredients, artificial ingredients, or anything that you cannot pronounce!

- Choose the most natural foods possible, such as 100% pure fruit juice and 100% whole grains. Avoid all processed foods and get meat and fish direct from the counter. If you desire added sugar or salt, then adding it yourself will allow you to control exactly how much you are eating.

- Avoid shopping with your children. They are much more likely to be swayed by colourful and unique packaging and will probably hound you relentlessly until you succumb to their whim. The best way to stop your family from eating junk food is to not buy it in the first place.

- The perimeter of most stores is where the majority of the healthy produce is. By avoiding the central aisles as much as possible, you will also avoid the temptation of unhealthy snacks and ingredients.

**Nutritional and Ingredients Labels**

There have been arguments by many individuals for a number of years calling for simpler food labelling. Understanding the immense amount of jargon on labels can be difficult, especially when the guidelines as to what needs to be included on them are, in some cases, ambiguous. We have already established that when it comes to living a truly healthy lifestyle, knowledge really *is* power. Understanding food labels is another key part of being able to make healthy and informed food choices.

*How to read food labels*

Remember that the information given on food labels is based on a diet of around 2000 calories per day. If you are female, there is a very good chance that you will not be consuming this number of calories each day, particularly if you are actively trying to lose weight. The number of calories that you should be eating each day is also determined by your age, gender, weight, and the level of activity that you do during the day.

Begin with the serving information which can usually be found at the top of the label. This will tell you the total number of servings per container and what the correct portion size of the product should be.

The % DV (Daily Value), depicted on the label, shows you the percentage of each single nutrient in an individual serving compared to the recommended daily amount. As a guideline, if you are looking to reduce your intake of a specific nutrient; for example, sodium aka salt, then you should look for foods that are labelled with less than 5% DV. If you are planning on increasing more of a nutrient, such as fibre, then look for labels stating more than 20%.

The AHA has recommended that, based on a 2000 calorie diet, certain items should be limited. This includes a maximum of 11-13 grams of fat, as little trans fat as possible, and no more than 1'500mg of salt. When the nutrition label states that a food item contains 0g of trans fat, but you spy the term 'partially hydrogenated oil' in the ingredients list; this is a key indicator that the product does contain very small elements of trans fat – less than 0.5 per serving.

*Common labelling terms unravelled*

Natural or from natural ingredients.

Many products state that they are 'natural' or 'made from natural ingredients'. Many of us believe that if a product states that it is natural, then it must be healthy, nutritious, and low in things like fat, sugar, and salt. However, it should not be assumed that these items are healthy. What the term actually means is that the food is free from artificial flavours, colours, or man-made chemical preservatives. They are not processed, but you should still check the ingredients and nutritional information carefully to ensure that they are a healthy choice.

## Fresh

If a product is labelled as being 'fresh', then it has not been modified or altered, such as being frozen in order to increase its shelf life. Fresh foods typically have a short window of sale between production and expiration.

## Pure

The term 'pure' is another ambiguous label on food produce that can be misleading. It is similar to natural in that it is designed to make us think that the item is going to be good for us, although essentially an item can only truly be considered pure if it is a single food with no added ingredients whatsoever. For example, a jar labelled as 'pure coconut oil' should contain 100% coconut oil and nothing else. If you are unsure if your product is pure, then always check the ingredients list.

## Low fat

As we have already established, low fat does not necessarily mean that it is good for you with many food manufacturers compensating with adding sugar, salt, or other flavourings to keep their product tasting delicious.

## Reduced fat

Reduced fat labels can also be misleading and, if we are in hurry, they can seem like a straightforward way to cut some of the fat out of our diets. However, research shows that many products that market themselves as 'reduced fat' often had much greater levels of fat in them to begin with, far more so than another product in the same genre of food. The rule here, yet again, is to not make any assumptions, but check the label and see exactly how much fat per portion you are likely to be getting. You may find an alternative brand, promoted as normal fat, may actually have the equivalent or even less than the one sold with supposedly reduced levels.

## No added sugar or unsweetened

During Chapter 2, we looked at sugars and sweeteners and now might be a good time to refresh your memory as to the differences between refined and natural sugars. Many people mistakenly assume that products marketed as unsweetened or containing no added sugar are pretty much sugar free. Wrong! What it actually means is that additional sugar or sweeteners have not been added to the natural contents of the product. For example, a carton of orange juice may state that it has no added sugar – which is great – but it will still contain sugar that is naturally found in oranges. This is where the distinction between natural and refined sugars is important. Whilst we must still not overload on natural sugars, particularly in view of the health of our teeth, the foods that they are found in are also extremely healthy and packed with nutrients, minerals, antioxidants, and fibre that is crucial to maintain our healthy new lifestyle.

Sticking to foods that are as natural as possible will ensure that you minimise your intake of refined sugars and artificial sweeteners. If you are in any doubt, always check the ingredients list!

Home-made

The idea of a product being home-made immediately creates a feeling of warm, comforting meals. However, it has no bearing on its nutritional value or if it is or isn't being mass-produced. What it actually means is that it has been produced in a domestic kitchen, not a factory, but as even a domestic kitchen can churn our large batches of food, your jar of delicious home-made bolognaise could actually be a bulk-produced low quality item. If you want truly home-made food that you can guarantee will be good for you, then your best bet is to get your butt in the kitchen!

A good source of fibre

Many products market themselves as being a good source of fibre, which as we know is an essential nutrient for keeping our digestive system healthy. However, there is no guarantee that this fibre is derived from natural sources. Instead manufacturers are using something referred to as 'isolated fibres' which have been made from chicory root or the purified powders of poly-dextrose. As with all of the recommendations in this book, naturally occurring fibres are a much healthier choice.

## Made with real fruit

You would like to think that a fruit product is actually made with real fruit, but the percentage of fruit used in comparison to other ingredients can sometimes be extremely small. Some products also deliberately mislead customers by claiming to be made from a fruit that isn't actually used to make it whatsoever. For example, you would expect Betty Crocker's Strawberry Splash Fruit Gushers to be full of concentrated strawberry goodness, right? Wrong, in actual fact the product contains NO strawberries and is made using pear concentrate.

## Made with whole grains

Similarly, a product that claims that it is made with whole grains could be made with only 1% whole grains and can still legally be able to be sold with that label. Many products marketed in this way have unhealthy primary ingredients such as refined flour or sugars, so make sure you check all the packaging before making a purchase.

Unfortunately, lax labelling laws make it very easy for manufacturers to mislead us into thinking that their products are healthy, natural, and good for us to eat. Obviously, it is impossible to read every label in a supermarket, you would be there all day, but if each time you shop you compare two or three different products, you will soon get a feel for what the better food choices are.

# Eating right doesn't have to break the bank

A lot of the blame for the rise in obesity is directed towards the higher price tags that seem to accompany much of the healthy produce that we should be eating. In particular, organic items are considered by many to be a luxury purchase that is simply unobtainable for many of us. Whilst you may have to juggle your budget to reflect a slightly more expensive food shop each week, the benefits you will soon feel from your new healthy lifestyle will soon outweigh any financial implications. You may even find that with your new planning strategies you save money by not making impulse purchases, wasting food, or ordering takeaways. However, with that said, eating well doesn't have to break the bank. Here are our tips for keeping on track when on a budget.

- Buy unprocessed foods. Whole or unprocessed foods are actually often cheaper than processed alternatives as you do not have to pay for fancy modifications or packaging. They are more nutritious and allow you to have full control over what you are eating. Staple unprocessed foods that you should be buying each week include: frozen chicken breasts, cans of tuna, plain yoghurts, eggs, whole wheat pasta and rice, beans, oats, and olive oil. You should also stock up on an assortment of fruit and vegetables. Choose produce that is in season to help keep costs down.

- Buy cheap proteins such as turkey, chicken, fish, eggs, and cottage cheese. You need approximately one gram of protein per pound of your body weight every day to help build and maintain muscle. As we have already discovered, proteins are much better for you, keeping you feeling fuller for longer by taking longer to break down.

- Frozen fruits and vegetables are a great way to keep to your budget. They are often half the price of fresh equivalents and have an almost infinite shelf life when stored in the freezer. They are also pre-cut and cleaned so that they are very convenient to cook.

- Buy locally. Supporting your local farms, butchers, and other food producers is a great way to boost your local economy as well as your health. They may not always be cheaper, but they normally have tastier and better quality products, plus your money is going back into local business pockets rather than a huge manufacturing company.

- Drink water. Filtered water is the best thing that you can drink both for your health and for your wallet. One filter will clean approximately 40 gallons of water so the initial outlay is miles cheaper than bottled water or sodas.

- Stick to your plan! One of the biggest budgeting fails is making impulse purchases when you are in the store. If you really have poor willpower, then consider shopping online instead, that way you won't be tempted by colourful store displays of discounted products.

- Grow your own. If you have some outside space, it is very simple to start your own little home-grown venture. From growing herbs in window boxes to having a chicken coop in the yard, there are no limits to the amount of fresh food you can create for yourself; all it takes is a little patience and imagination. There are plenty of ideas available online to make the most of the space that you have.

We hope that you have found this chapter full of useful information and advice for how to tackle the supermarket shopping. We have looked at the importance of planning ahead and ensuring that we stick to it! We have taken a look at what we should and shouldn't be filling our shopping carts with and given you a few tips on how you can avoid being tempted by discounts and special offers. We have examined some of the jargon used in packaging and labels and how to decipher what it really means, and finally, we shared some ways in which you can still eat healthily when on a budget.

All this eating right won't mean a thing though if we don't get up and get moving. That's right; during Chapter 9, we are going to help you get active! We cannot stress the importance of exercise in your new lifestyle, but we also understand that not everybody is ready to start in the same place. Whether it is walking for ten minutes or cycling for ten miles each day, every movement counts. We are going to coach you through the next chapter one step at a time. Ready? Steady? Move!

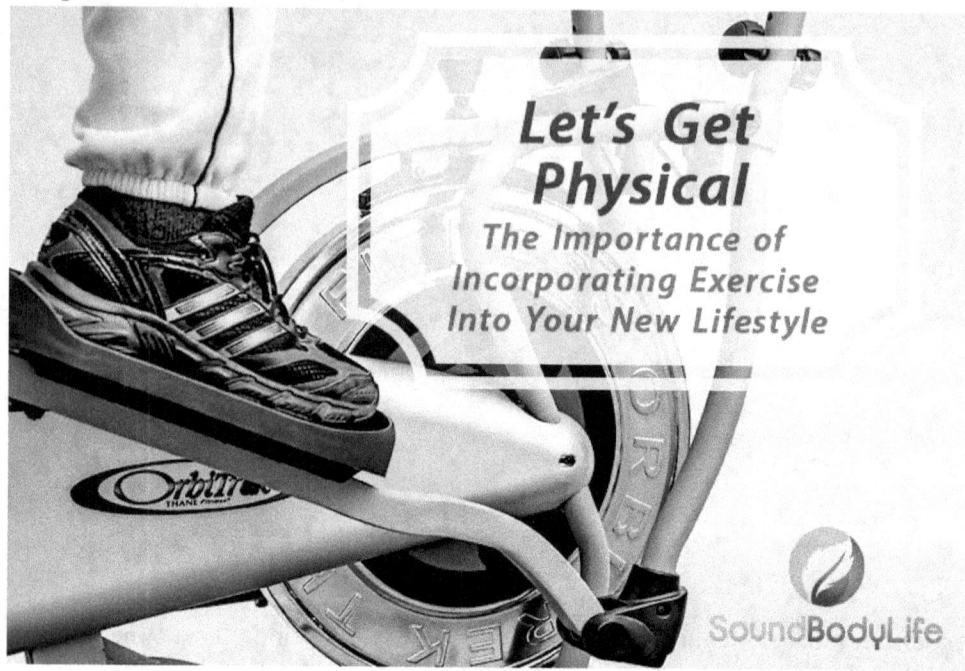

# Chapter 9

Let's Get
Physical
The Importance of
Incorporating Exercise
Into Your New Lifestyle

SoundBodyLife

Now that we know what food we need to be eating to fuel our bodies, it is time to get to burning that fuel. Diet is only half the battle when it comes to embracing a new healthy lifestyle. Getting up and getting moving is just as beneficial for losing weight and for your long term health. Even the smallest changes can make a difference, so what are you waiting for?

**The benefits of physical activity**

It truly is impossible to overstate the benefits of regular physical activity. Examples of ways that it can improve your health include:

- Controlling your weight.

Exercise, along with diet, is fundamental to controlling your weight. If you consume too many calories and don't burn enough of them during physical activity, then over time you will gain weight. How much exercise you need to do will vary depending on a number of factors including your gender, height, and current weight.

If you are looking to lose weight, then you will need to burn significantly more calories than you are consuming. There are many online tools that you can use to work out exactly how many calories per day you should eat to lose weight. Our favourite is: http://www.healthstatus.com/calculate/calories-to-lose-weight

- Reduce your risk of developing Type 2 diabetes and metabolic syndrome.

  Metabolic syndrome is a condition diagnosed by a person having high blood pressure, too much fat around the waist, high triglycerides, low HDL cholesterol, or high blood sugar. Type 2 diabetes is a result of our bodies not producing enough insulin or not using the supply effectively. Both are largely caused by unhealthy lifestyles. Research has shown that fewer people who exercise regularly are diagnosed with these conditions.

- Reduce your risk of cardiovascular disease.

  Just two and a half hours of moderate aerobic activity, such as brisk walking, can dramatically cut your risk of developing heart disease or having a stroke. Regularly participating in physical activity can also improve your cholesterol levels and lower your blood pressure.

- Reduce your risk of some cancers.

  Research has shown that physically active people are less likely to develop colon cancer than those who live a sedentary lifestyle. It also shows that women who exercise regularly have a lower risk of breast cancer. There has also been some evidence that suggests that an active lifestyle could potentially lower your risk of developing endometrial or lung cancer, although the research in these areas is not 100% conclusive at the time of writing this book.

- Improve your mental health and mood.

  Regular physical activity can support thinking, learning, judgement, and analysis, particularly as we age. It can also reduce the likelihood of developing depression or mood swings, owed to the release of endorphins, otherwise known as 'happy hormones,' provided by exercise. Studies have also suggested that exercise can help you get a better quality of sleep.

- Strengthen your muscles and bones.

  As we age, so does our muscular skeletal system, which basically holds our body together. Certain muscles and bones in particular are more likely to suffer time-related damage. Therefore, it is vital to do our best to protect our bones, muscles, and joints. Exercise can help us to do this.
  Moderate aerobic and toning exercises on a regular basis can help slow down the loss of bone density and help keep our muscles and joints flexible and efficient.
  Some scientific studies have shown that people who have regularly completed two to three hours of moderately aerobic exercise each week have a lower risk of hip fracture.

- Increase your chances of living longer

  Obviously, if moving more means a reduction in the chances of developing chronic and life-threatening conditions that claim too many victims far too soon, by increasing your physical activity you will also increase your chances of living longer.

Many people are put off by exercise in the belief that in order to make a difference, they need to spend hours and hours in a gym, or because they are afraid of looking silly or injuring themselves. However, we can tell you right now that none of that is the case. Brisk walking is safe for most people, can be incorporated into your daily life, and isn't the least bit silly.

However, if you are just starting out exercising, then the most important thing is to start slowly. Whilst episodes like cardiac arrests are very rare during physical activity, suddenly exerting your body when you have been used to a sedentary lifestyle can put unexpected strain on your heart and other muscles. So our advice is to start small and build up the time and intensity of your exercise gradually.

If you have a chronic health condition such as diabetes, arthritis, or heart disease, then you must consult with your doctor before undertaking any physical exertion. Your doctor will be able to advise you if your condition limits your ability to exercise and suggest how much physical activity you can reasonably and safely undertake.

**Get Walking**

The recommended amount of exercise for the standard American adult is 150 minutes of moderate aerobic exercise per week. You can break this down however you feel comfortable, but we suggest doing 30 minutes over five days of the week with the two resting days interspersed throughout your week. However, we realise that not everyone is going to be able to start at this level. If you feel that this will be too much exertion for you at first, try beginning with just ten minutes per day. The sooner you start, the quicker you will begin to reap the benefits and notice the difference, both in your weight and overall quality of health. If you are walking to lose weight, the UK National Health Service (NHS) states that just thirty minutes of walking will help a 60kg person burn off around 99 calories.

Walking is not only good for your health; it is also good for your wallet and the environment. The only energy that you will burn is your own and it won't cost you a cent. Plus, the only thing you will need is a comfortable pair of shoes. A recent report by the Ramblers and MacMillan Cancer Support entitled 'Walking Works' has explored the health benefits of walking and it found that 150 minutes of moderate to brisk walking each week could save 37'000 lives per year. It could also mean 300'000 fewer people each year are diagnosed with Type 2 diabetes.

Scientists at the Lawrence Berkeley National Laboratory in California believe that walking may even be more effective at reducing heart disease than running. They studied participants between 18 and 80 years of age over a six year period and the results showed that regular walking reduced the risk of heart disease by 9.3% compared to a reduction of only 4.5% seen in people who regularly ran.

**Walk this way**

The idea of walking may sound pretty simple to most of us, but in fact there are a number of things to take into account when we walk both to get the most out of the exercise and to protect our bodies.

The most important thing to consider when we begin walking is our posture. Engaging our core muscles is particularly important as we are upright the whole time, so we need to tighten those tummy muscles to properly balance our bodies and hold ourselves in the correct position. The best way to do this is to ensure that we stand up straight when we walk; shoulders back and no slouching. Keeping our chin parallel to the ground will also ensure that no additional strain is placed on the neck muscles. Try and relax your arms so that you aren't holding tension in them or your shoulders.

*Footwear*

As we have mentioned, having the correct footwear is the only piece of equipment you will need to start walking. However, with hundreds of different shoes on the market, how do you know what to look for? Here are our tips to help you source the correct footwear.

- Make sure that you wear the socks that you will be wearing for your walks or work outs when you go shopping. Also, remember that feet can swell up to half a size bigger during the course of the day, so go shopping towards the end of the day when your feet will be at their biggest. Doing both of these things can make a massive difference to the way that your shoes fit.

- You may want to consider specialist walking shoes. When we walk, we usually hit the ground heel first and most specialist walking shoes have a built in Achilles notch, which is a little dip down in the back of the shoes, in order to relieve pressure on the Achilles tendon.

- Try and opt for a shoe that is lightweight with breathable fabric. This will stop your feet from sweating too much. Also, try and pick shoes with a flexible sole that will move in harmony with your foot and ensure that your toes have room to wiggle and your heel doesn't slip.

- Give them a try. Many specialist footwear stores have treadmills or walking areas where you can try out the shoes to ensure that they are a good fit.

## Tracking your progress

One of the most common ways to track your progress now is by downloading one of the many apps that are available for your cell phone or other mobile devices. One of the best ones is the 'Map my Walk' app. There are pre-loaded routes in case you aren't sure the best way to walk locally to you or you can upload your own and see how much ground you have covered. You can also log the food that you eat and connect to social media to gain additional support and share your progress.

If you prefer a more traditional method of tracking, you can always purchase a pedometer and write down your distances in a notebook.

## Don't be scared to change it up

Once you have got used to walking regularly and can manage 30 minutes at a time, then changing your route can keep things fresh and interesting, thus keeping your motivation levels high. It will also avoid the inevitable plateau that comes when your body becomes too familiar with a routine. Some ways that you can add variety to your walks include:

- Do some speed walking. Alternate between regular brisk walking and speed walking, using a timer or certain benchmarks to tell you when to swap. Alternatively, if you listen to music whilst you walk, switch between the two after a certain number of songs.

- Walking uphill gives your gluteal muscles (buttocks) a serious workout. Walking uphill uses much more energy than on a flat surface and more energy = more calories burnt. If you are using a treadmill, just increase the incline to recreate the same movement.

- Give yourself an endurance test. Go for an extra long walk once a week.

- Change your route. Even walking your usual route from finish to start instead can count as a change.

With each walk, monitor how you feel afterwards to ensure that you are not pushing yourself too far. If you feel good, then you can always increase the length or the intensity the following week.

*Help the environment*

Walking is a positive step towards helping the environment by reducing the amount of pollution that is being released into the air. Short journeys should always be done on foot when possible as using the car for them uses almost twice the $CO_2$ per mile.

Researchers have also found that walking, particularly in green open spaces, can reduce your stress levels, improve your mood, and enhance your ability to concentrate and pay attention.

*Get your friends involved*

Another fantastic thing about walking is that anyone can do it with you. You can rope in your family, your friends, or your pet dog to go for a walk with you. You can still talk and enjoy one another's company, but you are getting fit and healthy at the same time.

There are also plenty of walking groups and associations with their details online, just check on your preferred search engine. If there isn't one where you currently live and you are quite sociable, then perhaps consider setting one up. There may be people just like you wanting to find other people to walk with.

The point is that you can walk solo or walk with friends; it is all beneficial for your long term health.

**How to get fit, whatever demographic you are in!**

Everyone leads busy lives. Whether you are a young person in school full time, a mother with a young family, or a little older with a job or active in your community, there are always things that can get in the way of exercising. The key is finding a way to incorporate it into your lifestyle so that it becomes routine. Here are our suggestions to get moving in your day to day life.

*Fitness for young people*

- Find a sport. There are always clubs and sports associations looking for new people to get involved. If you aren't sure what sport is for you, visit http://www.nhs.uk/Tools/Pages/olympics-sport.aspx which will give you a short psychological and aptitude test, developed by an expert team of sports psychologists at the UK's Loughborough University. It will then suggest which sport is right for you based upon the answers you have given.

- Do Couch to 5k. The Couch to 5k plan is a fantastic way to start running and build on your fitness. It begins with running in thirty second bursts with the aim that by the end of the programme you will be able to run for 5k without stopping. Find more information here: http://www.c25k.com/

- Walk more. From going to school to visiting your friends, aim for 10'000 steps every day.

- Find out if there is a local gym that you are able to join. Community centres often have gym equipment that you can use at a reduced cost. Just make sure you have a proper induction first.

- Get your mates involved too. Swimming, cycling, or skateboarding together can be great fun.

- Play interactive video games. Dance games for the Wii or Xbox can burn lots of energy and calories. Anything that gets your heart rate up is benefiting your health.

*Fitness for busy moms*

- Schedule in a time to exercise and stick to it. Straight after dropping the kids off at school works well as you are already up and moving.

- Walk your children to school. This will benefit their health too, and will save you money on gas.

- Split activities up during the day. Even doing three 10-minute work outs spaced throughout the day is beneficial.

- Utilise your waiting time. Moms spend a lot of time waiting – waiting for the microwave to ping, the iron to heat up, or the kettle to boil. Whilst you are waiting, do a dozen squats or calf raises. Alternatively, grab a couple of tin cans and use them as weights whilst you do some arm rotations. These moves may not burn many calories, but they will help with the toning and definition of your muscles.

- Get an exercise DVD. These are easy to follow routines that you can do in the comfort of your own home whilst the baby naps or the children are in school.

- Get active with the kids. Children love nothing better than running around outside. Get on their trampoline with them, take them swimming, or play some ball in the back yard. Every movement counts!

- Find a gym with a crèche. Many gyms now offer this service to encourage moms to use their facilities.

- Buggy up! Buggy-based fitness classes are extremely popular. Look online or in your local community magazines to see if there are any classes near you.


*Fitness for the whole family*
- Children who have physically fit parents as role models are much more likely to follow in their footsteps. Set a good example by encouraging as much physical activity as possible. It will also wear them out for bedtime!

- Spread the activities out during the day. It can be a lot to ask a small child to be active for a whole hour in one go. Instead break up the exercise into smaller increments during the day,: for example, start with 15 minutes on the trampoline and later do 15 minutes playing football in the backyard.

- Teach your child to ride their bike. Long cycling sessions are something that the whole family can enjoy together and are a fabulous way to boost fitness.

- Let your children decide how they want to get their exercise. Many children loathe physical education at school because they are told what sports they have to participate in. Giving them the choice means they will want to be actively involved.

- Go swimming. Almost all children love swimming and it is great for burning calories and toning muscles.

- Dance! Pop your favourite tunes on, turn them up loud, and encourage the whole family to have a dance around. It burns calories, is loads of fun, and the kids will love playing DJ.

## Fitness for office workers

- If you can, cycle to work. It is better for the environment, you won't struggle to park, and it is an easy way to incorporate exercise into your daily routine.

- If you cannot cycle to work, get off the bus a stop earlier or park the car a few streets further away. Even adding ten minutes of walking to and from your office will benefit your health.

- Visit people at their desks. With the introduction of emailing, calling, and even instant messaging, it is very easy to get lax about visiting other people's desks to speak to them. Sitting down for prolonged periods can actually damage your spine, so get up and walk over to them.

- Use your feet to go up and down floors. We don't just mean taking the stairs instead of the elevator either! If you have escalators in your building, walk up or down them instead of standing and waiting.

- Go out for a walk at lunchtime. It will also help clear your head and improve your concentration levels for when you return to work.

- If your office has a gym or your company offers corporate gym memberships, then take advantage. An hour for lunch is sufficient to have a bite to eat and spend twenty minutes on the cross trainer.

## Fitness for older adults (aged 65 plus)

- Try and incorporate movement into your daily activities. Light housework, gardening, and walking around whilst using the phone will all help keep your joints supple.

- Speed walking is a common physical activity for the older generation. Alternate between regular speed and rapid speed in order to sustain it for any period of time.

- Check your local community magazines and online to see if there are any local fitness classes that you can attend.

- Swimming is a great choice of physical activity for older bodies as the water helps support the body and relieves strain on the joints and muscles.

- Yoga is suitable for all ages and builds upon flexibility, strength, and balance. It is good to help you unwind and helps clear your mind and clarify focus.

- Tai Chi and Pilates are also ideal, low-impact exercises that you can do either in a class or from a DVD in the privacy of your own home.

## Those with physical disabilities

- There is no need to let physical disabilities hold you back from exercising. If you are able to walk, then walking is by far the easiest and most low-impact way to get started.

- There is also plenty of adapted equipment available online to help support you to reach your fitness goals.

- Other low impact exercises include yoga, tai chi, and pilates are good for reconditioning muscles and promoting healing.

- Again, swimming is ideal for those with physical disabilities as it does not put undue strain on the body.

## Now you have started – be consistent!

Consistency is the key to creating habits which we want to have in our new healthy lifestyle. We want to know when we are going to eat, when we are going to exercise, and how it is going to make us feel. After a month of being consistent, your new habits will begin to over-ride the old ones and before long you will not remember what it is to have an unhealthy, sedentary lifestyle.

Whilst we are aiming for complete and total health, it is also important to note that consistency of physical activity is vital for weight loss, too. It can be very easy to become bored and once you have missed one or two sessions it can be very hard to get back to regular exercise again. Here are our tips to help you be consistent in your routine.

- Start small. One of the biggest motivation killers for a new exercise plan is pushing yourself too much in the first initial days. You can end up aching for days or even injuring yourself, which will set back the progress. Instead, gradually build up the length and intensity of your workouts.

- Pick a space in your day and stick to it. Exercising at the same time every day will turn into a habit much more quickly and you can ensure that it fits around your time commitments.

- Find yourself a friend to workout with. Whether you go to a class, out for a jog, or do a DVD indoors, having a friend exercise with you can motivate you. Ongoing encouragement and support is vital to keep you on the right path.

- Vary your workouts so that you don't get bored. If you are going to an aerobic class one day, go swimming the next. Keeping your exercises varied will also ensure that you work different areas of your body.

- Do exercises that you enjoy. If you find the gym boring, search for a type of physical activity that interests you.

- Treat yourself to some new workout clothes or equipment. They can be huge motivation boosters as you want to try them out.

- Consider a personal trainer. PT's are great if you struggle with motivation or if you want guidance on specific exercises to achieve certain aesthetic goals such as toning up a wobbly stomach.

This chapter has been designed to help get you moving regardless of how much or how little exercise you have been doing previously. We have explained some of the health benefits that physical activity can bring and why it is so vital to your new healthy lifestyle. We have looked at why walking is the easiest exercise to start with and what you need to do to get started. Fitting exercise into our busy lifestyles can be a challenge and we hope that you find our tips on how to incorporate physical exercise into your daily routine useful. We would wish you luck with getting active, but we know you won't need it. You are ready and you can do it.

In the final chapter of this eBook, we are going to talk about keeping the changes we have implemented in place for the long haul. This is a sustainable lifestyle and we will help you keep motivated with a whole chapter of helpful information and resources. You've made the changes, now it's time to keep them – for good!

# Chapter 10

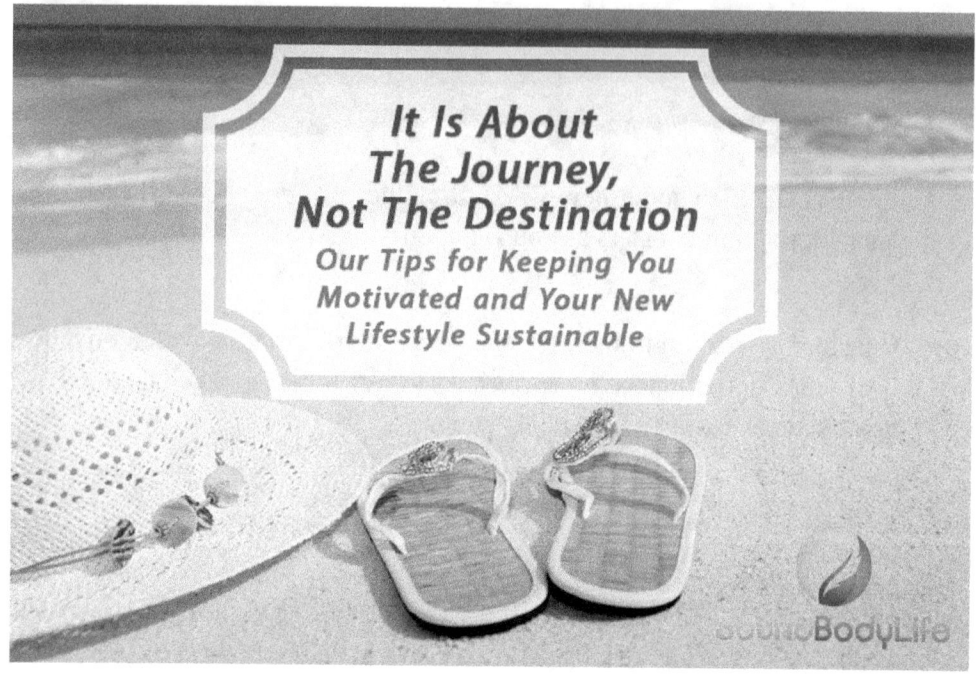

*It Is About
The Journey,
Not The Destination*

*Our Tips for Keeping You
Motivated and Your New
Lifestyle Sustainable*

'Do something for yourself today that your future self will thank you for'.

Welcome to the final chapter of this book and congratulations for making it this far. You now have all of the tools that you need to create a truly healthy lifestyle. During this chapter, we are going to look at the plans you can put in place to make this life a sustainable one.

Motivation usually comes more easily in the beginning. We are spurred on by the possibilities that are laid in front of us. In six months time, we could be slimmer, healthier, and have more energy than at any time in the last six years. Our dreams and goals drive us forward. We can picture that bikini body that we desire. We can see our health improving and our fitness levels soaring. However, we need to remember that there is no finish line for this lifestyle and in fact, it is actually sustaining this lifestyle that will prove to be the real challenge. Faced with constant temptation, it is all too easy to let one naughty food choice turn into a day of naughty food choices and then a whole weekend. The longer we are off the plan, the harder it is to get back on it.

However, there are things that we can do to help keep us motivated, assist us in getting back on track, and empower us on our journey to become healthier, fitter, and stronger human beings.

## Join a fitness group

The American Heart Foundation states that we are much more likely to stick to an exercise regime if we have company, so joining a fitness group could be extremely beneficial to your motivation. Lynne Vaughn, the Chief Innovation Officer of the national YMCA, believes that this is primarily because 'people don't want to let their buddy or group down' and so we feel obligated to exercise, even when we are tired and the sofa is calling our name.

There are hundreds of different groups ranging from running and hiking groups to baseball teams and zumba classes. One of the best things about going along to group fitness activities is that you can try them out and see if you enjoy them before making any sort of long term commitment. Many groups offer the first class completely free of charge too.

Group exercising also offers the benefit of socialization and friendship. This may seem daunting at first, particularly if you lack confidence, but being part of a group can help you create new bonds with like-minded individuals who can provide support and encouragement.

Exercising in a group can have a number of benefits including:

- Spending time with friends or family. With such busy lives, it can be hard to tie up a time to catch up with friends. However, by exercising with a friend, you can be sociable and raise your fitness levels in the same space on your schedule. Exercising with friends can also bring the fun factor into your workout, keeping it light hearted and enjoyable.

- Bringing out the competitive streak. Unless you are completely laid back, exercising in a group will automatically bring out your competitive streak. Be careful not to over exert yourself as this could cause injury, but a little competition acts as great motivation encouraging you to push yourself a little harder or for a little longer.

- You can support others, too. Whether you believe in karma or not, giving some support back to other group members can be beneficial for you as well as them. It will cement relationships and will enforce your position as a valued member of the group. People will also be more likely to offer you encouragement if you have already shown some to them.

Whilst group exercise is primarily a positive and effective way to improve your fitness levels and overall health, as with anything, there are a few things that, if not treated proactively, can potentially have a negative impact. If the group or class is too large, then you could feel anonymous and struggle to integrate with other members. You may need additional direction with any manoeuvres or exercises that you are unfamiliar with and, if the instructor has to get around a large class, you may not get the attention that you need. This also makes you more susceptible to injury. You are more likely to slack off in a class where the focus is so widespread.

To combat these issues, you can do a number of things. First of all, make sure you introduce yourself to your instructor or group leader at the start of the first session. A good instructor should then introduce you to the class and make sure that you are settled and check in with you regularly to ensure that you are able to follow the format for the session. If you have any concerns, then make your instructor or group leader aware so that they can assist you. They may well assume that you are okay unless you say otherwise. Finally, make sure you position yourself near the front of the group. This will help you get the leader's attention if you need it and make it easier to follow what is going on. You will also be less tempted to cheat or slack off.

**Make your new lifestyle a family affair**

Research shows that an individual who goes it alone in a lifestyle change where the rest of the family carry on as they did before is significantly more likely to fail. Support is everything and, if you can convince your family to embrace a more active and healthy way of living, then you can motivate and encourage one another. Before long, you will all feel the benefits that it can bring. So here are our tips for getting your family involved.

*Food for the family*

It can be very difficult to persuade some children to eat healthily, particularly if they have been primarily raised on convenience and processed foods. However, it is not too late to help them swap to healthier food.

- If they are resistant to vegetables in their meals, chop them very finely and mix them within dishes; such as cottage pie, spaghetti bolognaise, and enchiladas. This way you can get a lot of nutritious vegetables into them without them really noticing.
- Start small. You cannot expect them to make huge changes all at once either. Begin by introducing new fruits and vegetables one at a time. Swap to whole grain. Slowly reduce the amount of sugar in their tea or on their cereal. Gradual changes are a lot easier to accept and far less noticeable.
- When meal planning, get other family members involved. Find out what their favourite meals are and, if they aren't particularly healthy or nutritious, try and find a way to make them so. For example, if your kid's favourite food is pizza, then instead of buying frozen, make your own. Not only is it a fun experience to share with the family, but you are in control of the ingredients. You can opt for whole wheat pizza bases, low fat cheese, and vegetable toppings.
- Also, try and make some family rules regarding treats. One of the worst things that you can have in the house is a treat cupboard, as it becomes a massive temptation each time you walk in to the kitchen. Instead, suggest perhaps all going for a treat; such as ice cream once per week. It will give you time to bond as a family and make having the treat truly special.
- Now is also the time to educate your children in how to make healthy and nutritious choices so that they are equipped to make positive decisions regarding their food and eating habits as they get older and become independent. The level of learning you can share will depend on their age, but understanding where different food comes from, what types of food are processed, and what a portion size looks like are good places to start.
- Grow your own! This is another fun activity that you can involve the whole family in and is a great learning experience for younger children. You will have the added benefit of saving money and feeling safe in

knowing the exact origins of your produce. You can start as small as a window box or create a huge vegetable patch.

- Keep your fruit bowl well stocked. Ask each family member what their favourite fruit is so that they can always have a healthy and nutritious snack close at hand.
- Eat at the table together regularly. It may sound like an obvious suggestion, but huge numbers of people do not use or even have a dining room table. We understand that people have busy lives, but even scheduling one meal at the table together each week is important for family bonding and sets a fantastic example for your children to take forward.

*Get active together*

There are loads of fun activities that you can do as a family to help you get moving. Participating in physical activities as a family helps boost motivation and encourages kids to try out different sports and other pursuits. You will also be acting as a great role model. Studies have indicated that parents who spend more time with their kids are more likely to have kids that stay out of trouble. Getting them interested in sports and clubs at an early age can help encourage them to spend their leisure time wisely and keep them off the streets. Here are some ideas of things that you can do together.

- Walking. We have already looked at the benefits of walking, namely that it costs you nothing and anyone can get involved no matter how big or small you are. Whether you want to walk along the beach, through the woods, or even through a park in the city, walking is a great way to boost your fitness levels. It can also improve your mood and clear your head.
- Swimming. Almost all children adore swimming and it is a fantastic exercise. Learning to swim could save their life, so if you can teach your children or arrange for them to have lessons, then you will be providing them with a vital survival skill.
- Bowling is another pursuit that combines fun and fitness. It also teaches children about hand eye co-ordination and turn-taking.
- Baseball is a great sport that everyone can play at once. It combines cardio exercise with hand eye co-ordination and a competitive streak can make you push a little harder.

- Bike trips. When the weather is glorious it is an ideal time to get the family together for a bike trip. It can boost your fitness levels and improve your balance. Pack a healthy picnic to have at your destination and refuel you for the journey home.

## A few more motivational tips

- While there is no finish line for a healthy lifestyle, interim goals are hugely beneficial in marking your progress. Write down your ideals; such as 'lose 5kg,' 'be able to run for 3 minutes without stopping,' or 'cut out putting sugar in my coffee' and put them somewhere that you can see them all the time. Then put a great big black line through them when you smash them!
- Get an accountability partner. Even if you are mostly going it alone, find someone that you can 'check-in' with each week to keep them updated with your progress. This is one of the factors that work for a lot of slimming clubs. The idea that someone else is going to know if you have slacked off or cheated is sometimes too much to bear and can be a great motivator to stick to the plan.
- Keep photographs of yourself so that you can see your visible progress and remember that it is not all about losing weight. Other differences you will be able to physically see can involve toning up, better skin, and healthier looking hair and teeth.
- Remember to reward yourself, but keep it healthy! It could be a new book, a trip to the salon, or a new item of clothing, but remember that you have earned it and you deserve it.
- Have lots of sex! Yes, really! Not only is it physical exercise, but having an orgasm can release the same endorphins in your brain that eating chocolate does. Studies also show that even a 10% reduction in your weight can result in you having much better sex. As if we needed a reason!
- Raise money for charity. Making a promise that you are going to do something to raise money for a good cause can be a great way to keep your motivation high. There are plenty of charities that need your help and dozens of ways to raise money including: fun runs, sponsored swims, and, if you really want to push yourself, triathlons and marathons.

## Even if you are flying solo there is support for you

We understand that not everyone has a supportive family or friends. Flying solo deserves massive kudos in itself, as it can be significantly harder to get and stay motivated without the help of those around you. However, there *is* support out there for you if you are going it alone.

Here at SoundBodyLife, we are committed to embracing a healthy lifestyle that is in tune with our planet and we constantly work to live as naturally as possible. However, this wasn't always the case and having made the changes to this new way of life, we know exactly what you are going through now. With this in mind, we created our website www.soundbodylife.com in order to provide as much information and support as we can to people who wish to make the transition to greener and healthier living.

We strive to provide our readers with everything from instructions on how to make their own natural laundry products to how to embrace veganism. We look at nutrition, fitness, and overall health. Every article is full of the most comprehensive and relevant information that we can source to enable you to make informed decisions. We encourage our readers to participate in comments on articles and will always respond to any questions or queries that you may have. We are also happy to answer emails and if we do not have the answer you are looking for, we will do our best to point you in the right direction. Our promise to you is that we will always deliver clear, honest, and reliable information and recommendation on products and services.

Whilst you have reached the end of this book, you are still very much still on the journey to your new, healthy, and natural lifestyle. We hope that we have provided you with every piece of information that you could need to assist you in making informed choices and healthy decisions as you move forward. We have tried to be as comprehensive as possible, but if there is anything that you need further clarification on, please feel free to email the team at SoundBodyLife and we will do our very best to help you.

We wish you every success with implementing and sustaining the changes that you have decided to make. We have complete faith that you can do it.

And if at any time you are feeling that you can't go on, remember:

**'Nothing in the world is impossible if you want it enough. The word itself says I'm possible'.**

Get out there and do it.

**EXTRA RESOURCES**

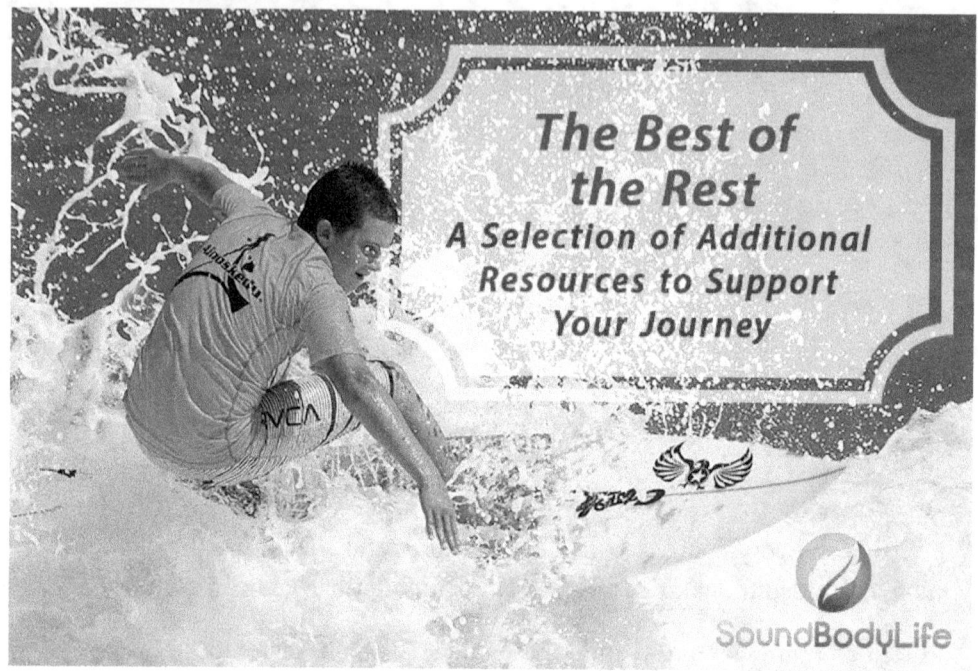

The Best of the Rest
A Selection of Additional Resources to Support Your Journey

SoundBodyLife

## OUR TOP TEN FAVOURITE COOKBOOKS

In no particular order, we are pleased to share with you our top ten cook books for healthy and nutritious eating.

1. The Natural Food Kitchen

Chef Jordan Bourke's book is packed with delicious and indulgent recipes that are also guilt-free, being made with natural ingredients and realistic alternatives to dairy, wheat, and sugar. With influences from around the world, this is one cook book you need to have in your kitchen.

2. Clean and Lean Diet Cookbook

By celebrity trainer James Duigan, this book is full of high protein meals that will leave you feeling fuller for longer. His one piece of advice for a healthy lifestyle is to avoid the C.R.A.P – caffeine, refined sugars, alcohol, and processed food.

3. Hummus Bros

As their name suggests, this chain of little eateries focuses on varieties of hummus. Their popular book educates the reader on how to make snacks, meals, and more with hummus and other influences from the Middle East.

4. Hemsley and Hemsley: The Art of Eating Well

We have all heard the phrase '*a little bit of what you fancy does you good*' and it certainly does in this cookbook. It allows a few naughty ingredients, but in sensible proportions that will not compromise your health. The recipes are straightforward and look utterly delicious.

5. The Medicinal Chef: Healthy Every Day

This fantastic book has recipes that are tailored towards a variety of health needs, including your immune system, heart health, digestive system, hair, skin, or joints and bones. Each recipe is easy to follow and could help improve your existing medical conditions.

## 6. Honestly Healthy Cleanse

Did you know that lemons are actually alkaline and not acidic? Well, if you didn't, that is just a sample of what you could learn from this book that is based on the principle of avoiding acidic foods that could irritate your system; including dairy, meat, and some grains. Its recipes are designed to cleanse and improve your digestive system.

## 7. Itsu: the Cookbook

Brought to you from the popular Japanese chain, every recipe in this book is less than 300 calories and takes no more than 30 minutes to make. They are packed full of flavour and ideal for a quick fix, low calorie dinner.

## 8. Plenty More

Although the recipes in Ottolenghi's vegetarian cookbook may appear complex, the majority of them are straightforward. A few unusual ingredients may leave you hunting beyond your grocery store for them, but the delicious recipes make it well worth the trip.

## 9. Total Greek Yoghurt Cookbook

This book by Chef Sophie Michell is inspired by her Greek heritage. In this book, she has designed some delicious and healthy recipes based around the use of Fage Total Greek Yoghurt, which is low in fat and high in protein to keep you feeling fuller for longer.

## 10. Green Kitchen Travels

As an extension of their health, travel, and veganism blog on greenkitchenstories.com, this latest book by the husband and wife duo David and Luise combines beautiful photography and delicious recipes, reflecting the different cultures and countries that have influenced them.

## OUR FAVOURITE NATURAL FOOD BRANDS

We are huge advocates of natural food brands. In no particular order, here are our favourites.

- **Rejuvenative Foods:** High quality fermented foods.
- **Kettle Chips:** There are some fantastic organic and vegetable varieties of kettle chips.
- **Tofurky:** Generally clean organic tofu products, avoid anything processed.
- **Mary's Gone Crackers:** Gluten-free, whole grain, and clean ingredients when snacking is a must.
- **Sunshine Burger:** Pretty much the only soy-free, wheat-free veggie burger option besides your own recipe. They may only do one thing, but they do it very well.
- **Field Roast:** Very clean mock-meats, but wheat-based and non-organic. Still, better than most else out there when you can't make your own.
- **Equal Exchange:** An emphasis on Fair Trade coffee and chocolate. Check ingredients on processed items.
- **Theo Chocolate:** They may not be vegan, but Theo's organic and Fair Trade varieties are a delicious option.
- **Artisana:** High quality clean nut butters in glass jars.
- **Bob's Redmill:** Stick with the solo ingredients rather than the mixes.
- **Dr. Bronner's:** They mostly make the world's best soap, but their coconut oil is now available in stores and it is by far the best-tasting Fair Trade coconut oil currently available.
- **Big Tree Farms:** A relative newcomer to the food industry, they are creating some revolutionary products, including coconut palm sugar. They also support farmers in Bali.
- **Traditional Medicinals:** Pharmacopeia grade herbs formulated by professional herbalists for high-quality, effective teas.
- **Nature's Path:** The go-to brand for organic cereal and a commitment to non-GMO ingredients. However, they do sometimes use a lot of sugar. So check the ingredients list of your product carefully before purchase.
- **Food for Life:** High quality sprouted grains.
- **Bragg's:** Amazing apple cider vinegar that you should incorporate into your daily diet.
- **Eden Foods:** Family owned business that use BPA-free cans, organic soy, no gelling agents in the soymilk, and have had a commitment to organic, local, and traditionally made foods for three decades.

## SOME OF OUR FAVOURITE RECIPES

Here is a selection of our favourite, nutritious, and healthy recipes to help get you started.

### Sexy Three Ingredient Smoothies

Each of these delicious smoothies has only three ingredients. Simple to make and packing a nutritious punch, they make an ideal breakfast or a filling and refreshing drink.

- **Strawberry Swing**

**Ingredients**: Strawberries, Yogurt, Shredded coconut

**How to:** Place 8 frozen strawberries, ½ cup plain kefir or pourable plain yogurt, and ½ cup shredded, unsweetened coconut into a blender. Blend until smooth. Makes one serving.

**Extras**: Spark it up with 2 tablespoons rolled oats, pinch ground cinnamon, 2 tablespoons flax meal, or protein powder.

- **Green Day**

**Ingredients:** Kale, Pineapple, Yogurt

**How to:** Place ½ cup frozen kale, ½ cup frozen pineapple, ½ cup plain kefir or pourable plain yogurt, and ¼ cup water into a blender. Blend until smooth. Makes one serving.

**Extras**: Add a pinch of cayenne pepper to freak this one out.

- **Caribbean Queen**

**Ingredients: Mango, Coconut Milk, Chia seeds**

**How to:** Place 8 pieces frozen mango (about ¾ cup) and ½ cup So Delicious coconut milk into a blender. Blend until smooth. Then add 1 tablespoon chia seeds and pulse just a few times to combine. Makes one serving.

**Extras**: You can add ground nutmeg, protein powder, or 2 tablespoons shredded, unsweetened coconut.

- **Bananarama**

**Ingredients:** Banana, Peanut Butter, Cacao Powder

**How to:** Place 1 peeled frozen banana, 2 tablespoons peanut or almond butter, 2 tablespoons cacao powder, and 1/3 cup water into a blender. Blend until smooth. Makes one serving.

**Extras**: Throw in protein powder, 2 tablespoons shredded, unsweetened coconut, a handful of raw almonds, pinch ground cinnamon, or 2 tablespoons rolled oats.

- **Not Easy Being Green**

**Ingredients:** Green Apple, Spinach, Ginger

**How to:** Place 1 green apple (with skin, cored, and cut into chunks), ½ cup frozen spinach, ½-inch piece peeled, fresh ginger (cut into small pieces), and ½ cup water into a blender. Blend until smooth. Serves one.

**Extras:** Blend in ½ of an avocado or fresh lime juice.

- **Channel Orange**

**Ingredients:** Bell pepper, Orange, Coconut Oil

**How to:** Place 1 red bell pepper (quartered, stem and seeds removed), 1 peeled navel orange, and 1 tablespoon coconut oil into a blender. Blend until smooth. Serves one.

**Extras:** Spice it up with cayenne pepper or ground cinnamon.

- **Blue Magic**

**Ingredients:** Blueberries, Almond Butter, Almond Milk

**How to:** Place ¾ cup frozen blueberries, 1 tablespoon almond butter, and ½ cup unsweetened almond milk into a blender. Blend until smooth. Serves one.

**Extras:** Add 2 tablespoons unsweetened, shredded coconut, a peeled frozen banana, 1 teaspoon pure vanilla extract, 2 tablespoons rolled oats, ½-inch piece peeled, fresh ginger, or 2 tablespoons flax meal.

- **La Isla Bonita**

**Ingredients:** Banana, Kale, Coconut Water

**How to:** Place 1 peeled frozen banana, ½ cup frozen kale, and ½ cup coconut water into a blender. Blend until smooth. Serves one.

**Extras:** Add a boost of protein powder, a handful of raw almonds, or ¼ cup frozen blueberries.

**MORE RECIPES**

**Spicy Chicken Stew**

**Ingredients**

2 leftover chicken breasts, cubed or torn into thin strips

4 C low sodium chicken broth

1 can diced, no salt added tomatoes, liquid included

1/4 C canned jalapeno peppers

1 small can corn, drained

3 cloves garlic, crushed

2 tsp cumin

1 tbsp chilli powder

1 tsp cocoa powder

**Directions:** Put everything into a big pot, stir, bring to a boil, then reduce the heat and simmer for 20 minutes uncovered, stirring occasionally.

**Serving Suggestion:** Eat with: Baked tortilla chips and guacamole: Peel and pit 3 avocados and mash along with 1 small onion, chopped; 2 Roma tomatoes, chopped; the juice of 1 lime; and 1 tsp salt.

**Nutritional Facts:** CALORIES: 427 CAL
**(Per Serving)**      FAT: 9.3 G
SATURATED FAT: 2.4 G
CHOLESTEROL: 94 MG
SODIUM: 966.7 MG
CARBOHYDRATES: 39.4 G
TOTAL SUGARS: 9.9 G
DIETARY FIBER: 6.6 G
PROTEIN: 50 G

# Potato Pancakes over Baby Greens

## Ingredients:

2 C leftover smashed new potatoes (1/2 recipe)

1/2 C liquid egg substitute

1/4 C finely chopped onion

1/4 tsp red pepper flakes

8 C baby greens

1 tbsp white wine vinegar

1 tbsp olive oil

1/2 tsp grainy Dijon mustard

1/2 C cherry tomatoes, halved

1/4 C freshly grated sharp cheddar cheese

## Directions:

1. In large bowl, combine potatoes, egg substitute, onion, and red pepper flakes.
2. Coat large non-stick skillet or griddle with cooking spray and heat to medium high. Spoon 1/4 cup mound of potato mixture onto hot pan. Repeat with 7 more mounds. Cook 15 minutes, turning once halfway through, until golden brown. (You may need to do this in batches, depending on the size of your skillet. Recoat pan with cooking spray in between batches.) Transfer to plate and keep warm.
3. Evenly divide greens among 4 serving plates. In medium bowl, whisk vinegar, oil, and mustard. Add tomatoes. Drizzle over greens. Top each plate with 2 pancakes and sprinkle with cheese.

**Nutritional Facts:**
**(Per Serving)**

CALORIES: 194.9 CAL
FAT: 8.7 G
SATURATED FAT: 3 G
CHOLESTEROL: 12.6 MG
SODIUM: 313.9 MG
CARBOHYDRATES: 21.1 G
TOTAL SUGARS: 3.9 G
DIETARY FIBER: 4.3 G
PROTEIN: 9.9 G

## Spinach and Spaghetti Frittata.

### Ingredients:

4 ounces whole grain angel hair pasta, cooked and drained

2 tablespoons olive oil

3 large eggs

3 large egg whites

2 tablespoons fat-free milk

2 tablespoons shredded parmesan cheese

1/4 teaspoon salt

1/4 teaspoon ground black pepper

1 package (10 ounces) frozen chopped spinach, thawed and squeezed dry

2 large plum tomatoes cut crosswise into thin slices

### Directions:

1. Preheat the oven to 375°F. With kitchen shears, cut the pasta into little pieces so it crisps more easily.
2. Warm the oil in a 10" ovenproof, non-stick skillet over medium-high heat. (If the skillet handle is not ovenproof, wrap it in heavy-duty foil.) Add the pasta and spread it out in the pan. Cook, turning often with a spatula and breaking up the clumps until the pasta starts to crisp, about 8 minutes.
3. Meanwhile, in a medium bowl, whisk the eggs, egg whites, milk, 1 tablespoon of the Parmesan, and the salt and pepper. Add the spinach, whisking to distribute evenly.
4. Pour the egg mixture into the skillet and reduce the heat. Cook for 2 minutes, until it firms up on the bottom; the mixture will be very green. Remove from the heat and arrange the tomatoes on the top. Sprinkle with the remaining 1 tablespoon Parmesan.
5. Transfer to the oven and bake about 10 minutes, until the eggs are set and the frittata puffs slightly. Cut into wedges to serve.

**Nutritional Facts:**  CALORIES: 276 CAL
**(Per Serving)**  FAT: 12 G
 SATURATED FAT: 2.5 G
 CHOLESTEROL: 160.6 MG

SODIUM: 398.1 MG
CARBOHYDRATES: 26.1 G
TOTAL SUGARS: 3.9 G
DIETARY FIBER: 3.8 G
PROTEIN: 14.2 G

**Easy Stir- Fry with Rice**

**Ingredients:**

2 tablespoons canola oil

1 onion, sliced

4 stalks celery hearts, chopped

2 carrots, chopped

1 clove garlic, minced

2 cups chopped bok choy

2 cups chopped mustard greens

8 ounces chopped cabbage and broccoli mix

4 scallions, chopped

3 drops hot-pepper sauce

2 cups cooked brown rice

Low-sodium soy sauce, to taste

**Directions:**

1. Heat the oil in a large skillet or wok over medium-high heat. Add the onion and cook, stirring constantly, for 2 minutes or until browned. Add the celery, carrots, and garlic. Cook, stirring constantly, for 4 minutes or until tender-crisp. Reduce the heat to medium- low. Add the bok choy, mustard greens, cabbage and broccoli mix, and scallions. Drizzle with hot-pepper sauce. Cook, stirring, for 5 minutes or until the greens are wilted.
2. Heat another large skillet coated with cooking spray over medium-high heat. Add the rice and cook, stirring occasionally, for 5 minutes or until lightly browned. Drizzle with soy sauce. Add the rice to the skillet with the vegetables and stir to combine. Cook, stirring frequently, for 4 minutes.

**Nutritional Facts:** CALORIES: 232.2 CAL

**(Per Serving)**

FAT: 8.3 G
SATURATED FAT: 0.8 G
CHOLESTEROL: 0 MG
SODIUM: 371.6 MG
CARBOHYDRATES: 35.6 G
TOTAL SUGARS: 6.2 G
DIETARY FIBER: 6.7 G
PROTEIN: 6 G

# Lemon- Scented Bread Pudding

## Ingredients:
8 ounces French or Italian bread, cut into cubes (5 1/2 cups)
1 1/2 cups light cream
1/2 cup sugar
1 tablespoon lemon peel
3 eggs
1 teaspoon vanilla extract
Fresh raspberries and/or blueberries

## Directions:
1. Grease a 9" x 5" loaf pan. Place the bread in the prepared pan.
2. In a small saucepan over low heat, combine the cream, sugar, and lemon peel. Cook, stirring occasionally, until the sugar is dissolved. Remove from the heat and let stand for 15 minutes.
3. In a large bowl, whisk together the eggs and vanilla extract. Slowly whisk in the cream mixture. Pour over the bread and press down lightly to make sure that all of the bread is moistened. Cover and refrigerate for 2 hours.
4. Preheat the oven to 350°F. Uncover the bread pudding and press down lightly on the bread to coat with filling. Bake for 35 minutes or until slightly puffed and set. If the top browns too quickly, cover with foil during the last 15 minutes of baking time. Cool on a rack for at least 20 minutes. Serve warm or cover and refrigerate for at least 3 hours. Serve with the berries.

**Nutritional Facts:**
**(Per Serving)**
CALORIES: 242.7 CAL
FAT: 11.6 G
SATURATED FAT: 6.2 G
CHOLESTEROL: 109 MG
SODIUM: 209.9 MG
CARBOHYDRATES: 28.9 G
TOTAL SUGARS: 13.2 G
DIETARY FIBER: 1 G
PROTEIN: 6.1 G

## EASY WEEKLY MEAL PLAN

### SUNDAY

*Breakfast:* Hot cereal: 2 servings of whole grain hot cereal. Top each serving with ½ cup of blueberries, 2 tbsp of toasted coconut and a tablespoon of walnuts. Have fresh fruit on the side.

*Lunch:* Roasted veggie and hummus wraps: Roast a pound of mushrooms, 3 bell peppers, and 2 quartered onions on a parchment-paper lined baking sheet in an oven at 400$^\theta$F. Cook until tender and browned. Chop into bite sized pieces once cool. Spread whole grain tortillas with hummus and fill with veggies. Put half the veggies aside to make the same again later in the week. Have a 100% sugar free popsicle for something sweet after.

*Dinner:* Carrot cashew spread on Woven Wheats, lentil chilli, and green salad: Warm up your lentil chilli. Have carrot cashew spread on Woven Wheat crackers on the side, along with a green salad made of romaine, carrots, red onion, and shredded cabbage. Have a healthy salad dressing on the side if desired.

## MONDAY

*Breakfast:* Apple-cinnamon Oat Squares: pack an Oat Square and a piece of fruit for a quick breakfast to start the week.

*Lunch:* Lentil chilli and salad with Orange Peanut dressing: pack lentil chilli, a big bag of chopped romaine, carrots, celery, broccoli florets, and roasted sweet potato. Pack a small container of Orange Peanut dressing and toss with the salad just before serving.

*Dinner:* Black Beans and Rice extravaganza: make half of the black beans and rice extravaganza recipe found here! Serve with a big side salad of lettuce, spinach, carrots, red onion, and healthy salad dressing. Have fresh fruit for dessert.

## TUESDAY

*Breakfast:* Green smoothie and whole grain English muffin with nut butter: blend 1 ½ cups of unsweetened non-dairy milk, 1 ½ cups of baby spinach, 1 ½ cups of frozen berries until smooth. Toast 2 whole grain English muffin halves and spread each with nut butter.

*Lunch:* Green pea guacamole wrap: Match a batch of green pea guacamole (recipe: here!). Spread whole grain tortillas with guacamole and top with sliced cucumber, shredded carrots, and sliced radishes. Roll up and serve. Have fresh fruit after.

*Dinner:* Cream curried cauliflower soup, roasted veggie couscous, and green salad: make a batch of cream curried cauliflower soup. Warm up your leftover roasted vegetables and serve over whole wheat couscous. Have a green salad of romaine, cabbage, celery, red onion, and healthy dressing. Save leftover soup for lunch.

## WEDNESDAY

*Breakfast:* Apple-cinnamon Oat Squares: pack an Oat Square and a piece of fruit for a quick breakfast to start the week.

*Lunch:* Garbanzo and veggie-stuffed pitas: Stir together a drained can of garbanzo beans, 2 cups of shredded lettuce, half a chopped avocado, 1 shredded carrot, 1 chopped cucumber, and 4 chopped green onions. Drizzle with tahini and orange juice and stuff into whole grain pitas. Have fresh fruit after.

*Dinner:* Romantic rice bowl: make a romantic rice bowl (recipe: here!) for two. For a vegan option, replace the chicken broth with water and substitute the chicken for Portobello mushrooms. Make a fresh fruit platter after using seasonal fruit.

## THURSDAY

*Breakfast:* Fruit smoothie and whole grain English muffin with nut butter: Blend together 2 cups of unsweetened non-dairy milk, 2 cups of fresh or frozen berries, and 2 tbsp of ground flaxseed. Toast 2 whole grain English muffin halves and spread each with nut butter.

*Lunch:* Cream curried cauliflower soup and romaine salad: have your leftover soup. Make a side salad of romaine, 1 chopped apple, 3 stalks of chopped celery, and 2 tbsp of chopped walnuts. Drizzle with orange juice.

*Dinner:* Whole grain pasta with greens and beans and green salad: Cook 12oz of pasta. Drain, reserving ½ cup of pasta water, and return pot over the heat. Toss with a can of white beans, 1 bunch chopped arugula, and a can of diced tomatoes. Add some reserved pasta cooking water if necessary to moisten. Save half leftover for lunch. Add a green salad of romaine, carrots, celery, broccoli, and healthy dressing. Have a fruit of your choice for dessert.

## FRIDAY

*Breakfast:* Hot cereal with dried fruit and nuts: cook 2 servings of whole grain hot cereal. Top each serving with chopped walnuts and raisins.

*Lunch:* Whole grain pasta with greens and beans with veggies: have last night's leftover pasta with a side of cucumber, bell peppers, carrot, and celery sticks. Fruit for dessert.

*Dinner:* Salmon or beans and wilted greens over Quinoa with roasted sweet potatoes: poach salmon in water and cook ½ cup of Quinoa. Cook some Swiss chard, spinach, or frozen greens until tender. Top with flaked salmon. For a veggie option, add cooked beans to the wilted greens and cook until heated through. Serve with Quinoa and roasted sweet potatoes on the side. Make a fresh fruit salad for dessert.

## SATURDAY:

*Breakfast:* Loaded English muffins & fruit salad: Cook a bunch of greens with a pint of halved cherry tomatoes and spoon over whole grain English muffins. Top with feta crumbles and serve fresh fruit on the side.

*Lunch:* Thaw some more of your lentil chilli and make a big salad of baby spinach, blueberries, carrots, radishes, and red onion. Make sure you use a healthy salad dressing.

*Dinner:* Make <u>vegetable enchiladas</u> and serve with a big green salad. Save any leftover enchilada for lunch the next day. Make <u>banana nice cream</u> for dessert.

# SHOPPING LIST

This shopping list will include all of the ingredients you need to make all of the foods on the above meal plan for two adults. The quantities are just estimates and you may want to increase or decrease them based on personal taste, any substitutions you may wish to make, or if you want to freeze anything for later consumption. You may want to divide the list into two shops to ensure you get the freshest ingredients, the choice is yours.

*Produce Fruits*

| | |
|---|---|
| 5 apples | 1 pint blueberries |
| 2 cups fresh/frozen berries of your choice | 2 bananas |
| 6 limes | 4 lemons |
| 22 servings of mixed fresh fruit for snacks and desserts | |

*Produce Vegetables*

| | |
|---|---|
| 1 bunch cilantro | 2 bunches green onions |
| 2 bunches radishes | 2 bunches arugula |
| 1 small cabbage | 2 bunches celery |
| 1 5lb bag carrots | 2 tomatoes |
| 1 pint cherry tomatoes | 6 hearts romaine lettuce |
| 2 bags of baby spinach | 1 small chunk fresh ginger |
| 1lb mushrooms | 2 cups fresh/frozen peas |
| 2 red bell peppers | 5 bell peppers (your choice of colour) |
| 4 cucumbers | 3 avocados |
| 4 sweet potatoes | 1lb broccoli |
| 1lb cauliflower | 4 yellow onions |
| 1 red onion | 2 heads garlic |

*Bulk*

These are items you will have to buy in packages containing more than you need, you can just use the amount in the recipes and keep leftover amounts for future use.

| | |
|---|---|
| ¼ tsp cayenne pepper | 3 tbsp salt-free chilli powder |
| 1 ½ tsp ground cinnamon | 5 tsp mild curry powder |

| | |
|---|---|
| ½ cup pecans | 1 cup raw cashews |
| 2 ½ cup walnuts | ¼ cup raw sunflower kernels |
| ½ cup and 2 tbsp shredded unsweetened coconut | ½ cup and 2 tbsp seedless raisins |
| 1 cup sesame seeds | 1 cup whole wheat couscous |
| 15 dried apricots | 1 cup pitted dates |
| ½ cup plus 2tbsp ground flaxseeds | |

*Grocery*

| | |
|---|---|
| 1 small bottle vanilla extract | 3 boxed unsweetened almond milk |
| 1 box unsweetened soymilk | 1 package steel cut oats |
| 1 package whole grain hot cereal | 1 box low sodium chicken broth |
| 2 boxes low sodium vegetable broth | 1 box of Woven Wheats |
| 1 16oz bag brown lentils | 1 16oz bag quinoa |
| 1 2lb bag brown rice | 2 cans no-added salt garbanzo beans |
| 2 cans no-added salt white beans | 1 can no-added salt black beans |
| 1 can no-added salt pinto beans | 1 jar tahini |
| 1 jar unsweetened peanut butter | 1 jar unsweetened cashew butter |
| 1 small bottle liquid aminos | 1 small bottle reduced sodium tamari soy sauce |
| 1 bottle rice vinegar | 1 can water chestnuts |
| 1 package sushi nori | 1 jar salsa |
| 12 oz whole wheat pasta | 4 15oz cans no-added salt diced tomatoes |
| 1 package whole grain English muffins | 2 whole grain pitas |
| 4 whole grain tortillas | 8 corn tortillas |

*Meat & Fish*

| | |
|---|---|
| ¼ lb fresh or frozen chicken tenderloins (for vegan option substitute for Portobello mushrooms) | 8oz salmon (for vegan option substitute for a can of no-added salt beans) |

*Refrigerated*

| | |
|---|---|
| 1 small tub barley miso | 1 half gallon orange juice |
| 1 tub of feta cheese crumbles or small chunk of feta | 1 small bag of part-skimmed shredded mozzarella |

*Frozen*

| 1 16oz bag frozen corn | 1 16oz bag frozen peas |
|---|---|
| 2 16oz bags frozen green blends | 1 16oz bag frozen bell pepper strips |
| 2 bags frozen berries | 1 box 100% fruit popsicles |

# USEFUL APPS FOR YOUR PHYSICAL MOVEMENT

Pact

Free to download on iOS and Android; Pact, formerly known as Gym Pact, is an app that challenges you to push yourself in your workouts by getting you to agree to a pact. The pact is simple. You agree to work out for a specific time frame on a specific number of days of the week. If you don't keep your side of the deal then you pay, literally. The minimum amount is $5 per day. However, if you keep your promise to work out, then you earn the same amount of money out of the pockets of other members who have failed to keep their pacts. The app is completely customisable, meaning that you can select how many days per week that you want to work out for, as well as how much you will pay each day.

Pact offers three different varieties of pact. A gym/exercise pact, a food logging pact, and finally a veggie pact. So how does it work? Well, the gym pact co-ordinates with your GPS and, to prove that you have worked out, you need to check in at your gym or leisure centre, or track your run using your GPS. Food logging is simpler and more forgiving as it just requires you to log all of your meals using the My Fitness Pal app. Similarly, the veggie pact asks you to upload photos of your veggie servings.

Whilst Pact may seem like a drastic way to encourage you to stick to your workout and healthy eating plans, if you are motivated by money, then it could potentially be the right app for you.

Fitocracy

Fitocracy is a social network just like Facebook or Twitter, except it is centred on fitness. Free to download on iOS and Android, it has full social media functionality such as status updates, profiles, and the ability to add friends. However, it is very game-orientated with each physical exercise you do earning you points and progress towards level-ups and badges.

This is a great app if you want to build up the support of an online community. Fitocracy has the option to cheer on your friends (similar to the Facebook 'like' button) and comment on their workouts. You can also get competitive with them for spots on certain leader boards.

## Runkeeper

If you are an avid runner or even if you are just starting out, then Runkeeper is the app for you. Also free to download on iOS and Android, it allows you to map courses via GPS, log your runs, set yourself goals, and track your progress. However, it is also a social network that lets you follow, train, and compete with those who you follow.

With custom leader boards, you can use your competitive streak to help motivate and encourage you. You can like and comment on your friend's runs and offer them support. You can also connect with your Facebook and Twitter accounts so that you can share running routes that work for you and let others know how you are progressing.

However, Runkeeper is not just for runners. You can log a variety of cardio workouts and utilise the goal-based training programmes that are available. The app is compatible with a number of third-party apps and accessories including Fitbits, Garmin GPS watches, and My Fitness Pal.

## BodySpace

BodySpace is a social network tied to BodyBuilding.com that is specifically geared towards weightlifters and is another app that is free to download on iOS and Android. It has all the functionality of an ordinary social network with features such as 'Fit Status' (status updates), a mood indicator that represents how motivated you are, and photo uploads. It also has the option to follow and friend people.

However, it is not purely a social media site. It also contains an exercise database, a workout programme database, and a link to the BodyBuilding.com store.

Whew! You made it! Congratulations!

I hope that you found the information provided here useful, and that it helps in your own weight loss journey.

In case you missed it earlier, don't forget to get your FREE BONUS by clicking the link below...

## SEND ME MY FREE BONUS NOW!

If you liked this book, or found the information helpful, please consider leaving a review on Amazon, I'd really appreciate it!

For more great info, make sure to check out the blog at www.soundbodylife.com.

Thanks!

Adam